Echo of Edith

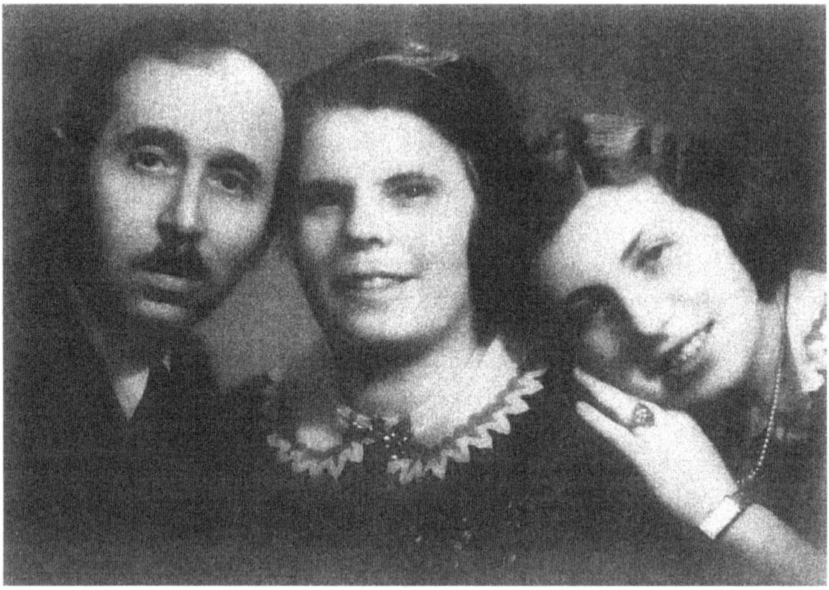

Hugo, Aranka, and Edith

Echo of Edith

Erwin K. Koranyi

GSPH

GENERAL STORE PUBLISHING HOUSE
499 O'Brien Road, Box 415
Renfrew, Ontario, Canada K7V 4A6
Telephone 1.613.432.7697 or 1.800.465.6072
www.gsph.com

ISBN 978-1-926962-53-5

Cover art, design, formatting: Magdalene Carson
Printed by Custom Printers of Renfrew Ltd., Renfrew, Ontario
Printed and bound in Canada

Library and Archives Canada Cataloguing in Publication
Koranyi, Erwin K
Echo of Edith / Erwin Koranyi.
ISBN 978-1-926962-53-5
1. Bock, Edith, 1916-1942. 2. Holocaust, Jewish (1939-1945)--Hungary--Biography. 3. Auschwitz (Concentration camp)--Biography. 4. Medical personnel--Hungary--Biography.
I. Title.
DS135.H93B63 2012 940.53'18092 C2012-901903-8

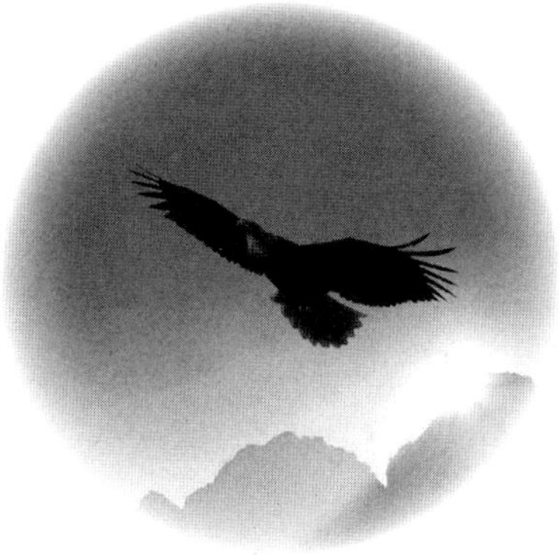

Acknowledgments

I wish to thank my good friends Heather Raff, Ph.D., Judith Stoller, and Professor Ann-Barbara Graff, Ph.D., for reading my early manuscript and providing useful suggestions and encouragement. I am most grateful for that.

I want to thank my senior editor, Jane Karchmar, who evaluated my writing, finding it a "powerful story." She worked on it with devotion and did a wonderful job of making it fly.

I also wish to express my appreciation to Magdalene Carson, artist, and the designer of the imaginative cover and layout of this book. And I thank the staff of General Store Publishing House.

CHAPTER ONE

The simple rented room, located in the student district in a venerable old apartment building with a trace of mouldy odour, became Edith's new home. Her landlady, Jolana, probably in her early sixties, regularly rented rooms to students for money and friendly company and was more like an aunty for Edith. Prague was an unknown city to Edith, and student life, away from her cozy home, a strange new experience. It was late October 1934. Barely five months had passed since Edith had graduated with honours from her high school in her small hometown, Zilina, which had been her world up to now. Zilina was in northern Slovakia, located at the foot of the mighty Tatra Mountain, on the right shore of the clear, ice-cold waters of the Vah River that cascaded down past the pine forests from the snow-covered peaks.

Edith had arrived in Prague at the end of August and had registered for the first semester of medical school at the ancient German University, recently split from its twin, the Czech-speaking Charles University. She had been excited to come to this lively city, bursting with intellectual and cultural life, music, commerce, politics, and science. All these now became her tempting future — a challenging, inviting, but also rather frightening proposition for a young girl who was for the first time away from her family.

It was convenient for Edith to follow the earlier set plan and to return briefly to the cushiness of her immediate and extended family in Zilina, and to the accustomed, amicable neighbourhood of her childhood. The Jewish high holidays were coming, always observed festively together at the New Synagogue and led by Rabbi David Friedman. The entire Bock and Kohn family participated in the services. Besides, the birthdays of all three Bock children fell so close to one another that it was handy to celebrate them all on one single appointed day: Edith's eighteenth; and the two boys, Laci and Zolo, were turning fifteen and fourteen, respectively.

Edith was a tall, shapely, chosen-to-be-blonde, young woman with attractive features, a sharp mind, and an effervescent nature. She always was the most popular among the large family, and with numerous friends and swarming boyfriends.

With tears in her eyes, Edith recalled the last of the family dinners. At the festive Friday evening meal, with head and face covered with a delicate scarf, Edith's mother, Aranka, lights the candles, her hand slowly circling the yellow, flickering flames; Hugo, her father, wearing *kipa*, blesses the bread and wine with ancient Hebrew chants. The entire family venerated the Sabbath, but even more precious was the customary togetherness of the family. Without Edith's presence, the weekly family experience would change now forever.

Then, too soon, back to the familiar, mustard-coloured railway station where she boarded the rhythmically puffing steam-train with all those red-capped railway workers blowing their whistles and waving their multicoloured lights; mother smiling and wiping her tears with her white hankie; a sullen father stuffing some extra cash in Edith's pocket; and Edith feeling guilty as the train, steam blowing, slowly set into motion toward an unknown future.

Now, back in Prague once again, Edith sat in front of her mirror, examining her face. Her thick, somewhat curly honey-blonde hair embraced her face, her pleasant, girlish features, and her sharp, dark eyes that looked back at her, while she applied a dab of light pink lipstick and inspected her narrow, plucked, pencil-darkened eyebrows. She did not put on any makeup and even removed the fashionable "half-moon lacquered" nail polish, leaving her nails plain and natural.

Yes, the recent holidays were wonderful but had passed too speedily. Her mother, Aranka, a skilled seamstress, had made for Edith a new outfit, her birthday present, and Father had given her a new wristwatch. The new black outfit had practical lines: a snug skirt, the hem covering her calf with a split between the knees, permitting free movement. The long-sleeved jacket was tightly fit with slightly padded shoulders. A simple white blouse completed the fashionable costume, feminine and practical, just what she needed for her student days.

How did Mother know what to make? wondered Edith. But then she was aware that Aranka had worked as a dressmaker at their modest home in the earlier part of their marriage, when her father, Hugo, had just begun his by now successful retail and wholesale toy store. Those were the Depression years, before they built the new family home. The expensive Swiss watch father had bought her as a gift had a second hand "to count patients' pulses," a somewhat premature notion.

Edith worried about Father: he had lost weight, joked less, smoked more cigars, and his temples had turned silvery. What was bothering him? Business? No. Maybe what Rabbi Friedman was preaching on the holidays, the "modern-day Haman," meaning the previous year's political changes taking place in Germany, when Hitler had come to power? She dismissed that idea, too. Nothing to fear, Czechoslovakia had a strong, modern army and was covered by treaties to the east and west. Her experienced, mature leadership was well respected internationally. What is Father worrying about, then? *Because I am leaving the tight-knit family for Prague?* thought Edith. That must be it! She recalled the family outing to the nearby Strecno Castle, Father driving his large, convertible Tatra automobile . . . the family picnic . . . the good time they all had . . . almost as good as picnics they had had many times before. She once again enjoyed seeing the silent ruins of the romantic old Gothic castle, keeping its unspoken secrets.

It was good to see the boys, too. Neither of the two, Laci and Zolo, were great students but they had wide interests and skills. Laci was quite artistic; his handwriting was as good as if it were printed. He could paint lovely pictures with oils; he could sew, knit, and was very handy; he had taught himself to play the violin and the trumpet. Zolo was more interested in mechanics and motors. Joseph was the youngest of the Kohn brothers, Mother's youngest brother, actually an uncle, but he was hanging around most of the time. For Edith he was more like one of the guys.

It was very early, just past six a.m. Still dressed in her sheer slip with narrow shoulder straps, in her underwear and the silk stockings she so loved, fastened by clips, Edith quickly put on a housecoat, went to the kitchen, and prepared some strong coffee. That was her breakfast: two cups of coffee, one with a plain bun, the other with a cigarette. Edith was not a smoker before, but all her girlfriends, not to mention the boys with whom they flirted, were smokers, puffing away in luncheonettes, coffee houses, everywhere. The air was always milky blue, smelling of bitter cigarette fumes, so Edith, defensively, started to smoke; then, of course, she got hooked. Now smoking had become a necessity.

She rushed back to her room, put her dress on, took one more look in the mirror, a touch of adjustment, patted her hair. She grabbed her coat, gloves, handbag, and a small leather case with notebook, paper, and a fountain pen; she also took her navy hat, a compromise, since she hated hats. She ran down the still empty staircase and onto the awakening street, automobiles competing with noisy streetcars, horse-drawn coaches with horse's hooves clicking, humanity rushing, swirling in different directions.

She was sure that she would be the first to arrive. This was the reason why she got up so early in the first place. The nearer she got to the university, the larger the student crowd became. She found herself in front of a gloomy, grey building, the "*questura*," as it was called in all European universities — Latin for "administration." She was impatient because she did not want to miss the first lecture of Professor Otto Grosser, the head of the Anatomy Department, and also Rector of the German University. But no choice.

A girl beside her in the lineup, also a first-year medical student, Helene Marek, turned to her. "Where are you from?"

"Zilina, and you?"

"From Bratislava"

"Also medical student?"

"Like you."

"There are not too many girls in the class."

"I would not expect it."

"Your outfit is lovely—must have been expensive; where did you buy it?"

"My mother made it."

"Lucky you," said Helene. "Maybe I shall travel to Zilina."

Finally, it was Edith's turn to pay the fee and obtain the rubber stamps in her official Report Book. She arrived at the lecture hall at just five minutes to eight.

The lecture was scheduled for 8:00 a.m. and started precisely, by the second, fifteen minutes later: the famous "*Academische Firtle*," the "academic quarter" (a fifteen-minute grace period before an academic lecture).

Professor Grosser, dressed in the requisite black coat with red decorations, began talking in a very clear and loud voice. He was known to be a superb lecturer, carefully explaining every single detail in an unambiguous manner, and never repeating himself. Thereafter, he demanded perfect knowledge of the subject. He was known, unlike the rest of the professors, unexpectedly to summon a student or two from the audience and confront them with a question about something he had taught earlier. Consequently, everyone burned the midnight candle, never allowing unlearned material to accumulate. On examinations: colloquia, rigorosum, Professor Grosser was merciless. Yet, everyone liked him.

"Anatomy is the soul of medicine, and some of you gentleman and alas! ladies as well, may even make it. Anatomy, physiology, and pathology are the preconditions to achieve your dream and become a physician. It happens to be my responsibility to teach you all anatomy, topographic anatomy, and dissections to perfection. Nothing less will do. You have seen the painting by Leonardo Da Vinci, who was a great anatomist, and Rembrandt's *The Anatomy Lesson of Dr.*

Nicolaes Tulp in The Hague. So, if you can't hack medicine, you always can take up painting.

"Dissection happened to be an ancient art which at one time had to be done secretly because of Church rules. It may even have started, shocking! with vivisection. Aristoteles inherited from his physician father an interest in the human body. Contemplating the human soul, Aristoteles came to the conclusion that the soul is a 'burning flame within the chest cavity which extinguishes when the person dies. So, there is no proof to it,' said the master philosopher.

"But one of his practical-minded teenage students interrupted him: 'Simple, Master. Just get a condemned criminal from the jail and cut his chest open while he is still alive, and look,' suggested the young man, who later became known as Alexander the Great, whose goal was to conquer and unify the entire known world. He came close to it but died at the young age of thirty-three. One of his generals, Ptolemaius of Egypt, built the town Alexandria, to remember his master, and also raised the amazing Alexandria Library and University, pride of ancient times. And there, Alexander the Great's suggestion came to reality.

"How do we know this? Aulus Cornelius Celsus, in his book of the second century, *De Medicina*—which was obligatory reading in the original Latin when I was a medical student—says: '*optima facisse*,' best way it was done by '*Herophilius et Eraristratus, qui nocentes homines a regibus ex carcere acceptos*,' who obtained condemned humans with the king's permission from the jail '*vivos inciderint*,' and cut them open alive . . .

"But anatomy has progressed since then. Andreas Vesalius's work *De Humani Corporis Fabrica* in 1543 corrected the anatomic mistakes of Galenus. The publication almost did cost him his life for opposing the Church's dogma; but he launched what we call the modern anatomy. In the same year, 1543, the work of Nicolas Copernicus, *De Revolutionibus Orbitum Coelestum*, was published. For that reason, most historians regard the year 1543 as the end of the Middle Ages. If you want to make an investment in your future, buy yourself the *Anatomy Atlas* of

Sobotta. It is expensive; so you may value it more. See you tomorrow in the dissection room."

The lecture of Carl Cori had been cancelled, for he had not arrived from Graz, Austria, where he was engaged full time as Professor of Physiology. In Prague, he had agreed to be only a guest lecturer, and the course was provided mostly by his assistant. Cori was an exceptional researcher on carbohydrate metabolism, working together with his Jewish wife, Gerti, no lesser talent than his own. (Eventually the two shared the Nobel Prize for the famous Cori Cycle.) His arrival was rescheduled for the day after next.

On her way out, Edith bumped into Helene Marek again.

"Just as well that the presentation was postponed," said Helena. "I am starving."

All over Europe, lunch was the traditional main meal, with three courses. Even the stores closed down for two hours at lunchtime.

"Me, too. Where are you having lunch?" asked Edith.

"Around the corner is a small restaurant, the Domoj, with good enough Czech food and it is cheap, too."

"Let's go there," responded Edith.

Indeed, the place was close by. As they entered, the air was heavy with the smell of onions and cigarette smoke. There were no empty tables, but they got two seats at a large table where four students were about finished eating. They were Markus Pavel, a second-year medical student; Klara Novak, a third-year philosophy major; and Teresa Janovic and Gisella Herzikova, both political science students. A weary, sweaty young waitress who was known by her first name only, Irene, circled the room.

"What's the special for today?" asked Helene.

"Green pea soup and pasta pockets filled with plum marmalade; no meat today." Both Helene and Edith ordered the same.

The four at the same table had already finished eating and lit cigarettes and continued their discussion.

"I read *The Trial* twice very carefully," said Gisella. "Don't tell me otherwise — the man is crazy. I mean mentally ill."

"Craziness has nothing to do with it," remarked Klara Novak, the philosophy major. "When Thomas Mann lent Kafka's book to Albert Einstein, the two of them met, you know, at Berta Fanta's place, for Einstein was teaching at our university at the time. Einstein shared your opinion. Unfortunately, Kafka has been dead for ten years now, so we cannot summon him. But he surely would have had to be more than just crazy, otherwise he would certainly not have been a welcome guest at Berta Fanta's very elite Tuesday night gatherings and literary circle. Martin Buber and similar characters were regulars. Einstein used to go there bringing his violin — "

"I like Kafka," interrupted Edith, "but first you must grasp his warped world. To me, *The Trial*, with all its participants, is the tragedy dwelling within Kafka's own brain. The main character, 'Mr. K.,' is the thinly disguised accused, Kafka himself, with his ubiquitous, devastating guilt. The lawyers, the arresting officers, the presiding judge in the book, all are the different parts of Kafka's own psyche, at war with one another. Did you notice, he always writes about the same thing: guilt, punishment, execution, about himself, like in his short novel *In the Penal Colony*.

"Peculiar? Surely. Kafka's father was a corpulent and rich man; Franz was slim and, though a Doctor of Law, he barely made a living. His father did not hide his contempt of Franz. Several of Franz's siblings died in infancy, but he survived. He never could maintain a normal sexual life. He preferred 'one-night stands' with simple girls or prostitutes but loved brilliant women asexually. He was also a vegetarian, like all of us today at this meatless lunch." Edith fell silent.

"A peculiar, challenging view but certainly not without sense," said Klara. "It reminds me of Sigmund Freud." Klara obviously valued Freud, particularly his philosophical views laid down in his book *The Future of an Illusion*. It earned him the Goethe Prize of Literature in 1930.

"Yet, to me, it is the threatening milieu of some kind of an approaching, cruel dictatorship, threatening all of us. That is what Kafka writes about," said Helene.

"You mean, Edith, your concept is something like the limbic system of the brain that Papez, the neuropsychologist, is writing about nowadays?" questioned Marcus Pavel.

"I still have not worked out the details," said Edith. "But the dark side of human nature certainly is our heritage since ancient times."

The pea soup was good but cold. *And Mother makes much better jam-filled pockets*, thought Edith.

"Yes, yes, the little country girl from Zilina," remarked Helene when they left, giving Edith an affectionate hug. "Are you Jewish?"

"Yes, I am. And you?"

"Me, too." The two started to giggle.

CHAPTER TWO

There was no trace of Professor Otto Grosser, but a veritable little army of anatomy demonstrators received the students in the huge, brilliantly lit dissection hall, where spoken words tended to echo and play tricks with one's mind. There were fourteen grey marble blocks or tables, seven on each side of the hall, all equipped with a shiny water faucet, sprinkler, and sink. On each of them lay a naked, stiff, cold cadaver, as grey as the marble blocks, mostly males, some females. They had long ago lost their human semblance and become specimens. Rubber-gloved, white coat-clad, the hesitant students lined up, four of them at each cadaver. Half of the students were working on the arms, the other half on the legs. Shiny surgical knives, scissors, forceps, and probes were laid out in front of each student.

The air was heavy and dizzying with the penetrating chemical smell of formaldehyde, which made their eyes tear up. A straight cut had to be made on the skin, leaving behind a clear, slightly oozing, red line. Obeying the instructions, the cut surface of the skin had to be grasped with the forceps, lifted, and freed from the under-surface. That done, the area opened up like a rose—but it did not smell like a rose at all. A strange, unpleasant, stale odour of death, mingled with formaldehyde, oozed throughout the room. The corpse on which Edith worked was an elderly female. Edith's hand shook slightly as she hesitantly made her first cut. She heard some of the boys at the neighbouring table laughing, evidently making tasteless fun of the corpse, attempting to overcome their own confused emotions with bravado. They were sharply reprimanded by the demonstrator. Edith was overtaken by a strange emotion but she concentrated on the task at hand.

"The cut must be straight, penetrating the skin, but don't dare to damage the muscles. You clean away the vessels, the subcutaneous tissues, the fascia, but, heaven forbid, don't dare to cut the nerves. Capital punishment, you know."

Now Edith, with her scissors, loosened the under-surface of the skin, on both sides of the incision. (*Was she right-handed? Did she like to knit?*) Some yellowish fluid appeared — lymphatic fluid. Edith cleared away the lymph nodes and wiped clean the surface. (*Did those arms ever hold a baby or grandchild?*)

"You are dreaming! Are you well?" raised the voice of the demonstrator. "Girls often faint in the beginning, you know. Not a bad job so far," and he walked away.

Edith tried to dismiss those personal thoughts about the corpse, and she now concentrated on her work until she was interrupted again by a commotion and mingling of voices and noises. Somebody had fainted. Good heavens, was it Helene? No, it was one of the boys. Edith felt relieved. She could not repress a gratified smile.

Edith worked now with determination. She laid open the complexities of the triceps and biceps muscles. At one point, she held the radial nerve in her forceps, believing it to be a blood vessel, and was ready to cut it away — but the forceps slipped at the last moment. It was then that she realized what the structure actually was. So, thanks to the near accident, she did a perfect job.

The inspecting demonstrator was pleased with Edith's work. "Where did you learn to dissect like that?"

Edith shrugged her shoulders but did not say that she used to cut up the chickens for the Sabbath dinners. (All vessels and all traces of blood had to be cleaned away to make the meat "kosher.") Just then, Professor Otto Grosser walked by, looking for the demonstrator. He paused for a few seconds behind Edith and bent down and looked at her work. "What is your name?"

"Edith Bock."

"Hmm," he said. According to the demonstrators, that was the highest level of recognition.

Later, Edith had the opportunity to discuss with Helene her fear of Helene's "fainting" and her relief that it was not her friend who had collapsed. Helene laughed heartily. They were at the little Domoj restaurant, and Irene, the waitress, took their order for the specialty of the day: mushroom soup and beef goulash. The goulash was quite good, but the mushroom soup a disappointment, compared to what she was accustomed to eating in Zilina.

At the next table, three students wrapped in cigarette smoke were immersed in serious political debate. Helene and Edith listened attentively but did not take part in the discussion.

"Things are coming to a head, man, I am telling you. Just watch the accumulation of the events in the last two years. Hitler succeeded in manipulating the good old president, Paul von Hindenburg, to appoint him as Reich Chancellor in January 1933. Hitler wanted Hindenburg to pass emergency laws against communists but he did not succeed. Soon after, in February, a communist Dutchman, Marinus Van der Lubbe, set fire to the Reichstag — that is the Parliament building in Berlin. Pretending outrage, Hitler privately called it a heaven-sent gift. The Emergency Law was passed, and communists, including communist Members of Parliament, were arrested for treason.

"Hitler, in the past ten years, has built the SA, the Brown Shirts, a conglomeration of hoodlums, by now some two million of them, under the command of Ernst Röhm to do all the dirty work Hitler needed. Opposing the SA, he also created the SS under Heinrich Himmler. The SA, which had helped him all along, firmly believed in socialism, if not communism, which was included in the official name of the party: Deutsche Nazionalsocialistische Arbeiter Partei — briefly, Nazi party.

"In late July of this year, using the SS, 'The Night of the Long Knives' was set in motion. The unsuspecting Ernst Röhm and the entire SA leadership were murdered in one single, blood-soaked night, and the rank-and-file troops came under the authority of the army. Then the entire army had to swear unquestioning obedience and loyalty personally to Hitler. One month later, just four months ago, Hindenburg died, and Hitler did not hesitate to assume the presidency as well, thus transforming the Weimar democracy to a dictatorship. He became 'Der Führer.' "

"And the until then pro-Czech Sudetendeutsch Heimatfront, the DNSAP, was dissolved. In its place, the Sudetendeutsch Party, the SdP, came into existence under Konrad Heinlein — "

"But Heinlein made solemn pro-Czechoslovak speeches — "

"Just watch him be transformed into an enthusiastic Nazi when the time comes — "

"Not only that, Hitler made a ten-year alliance with Poland this year, declaring cordial relations with them for ten years — "

"Oh, his foreign policy! Hitler made an attempt in July 1934 via the Austrian Nazi Party to take over Austria. When he failed because of Austrian prime minister Engelbert Dollfuss's resistance, Hitler had him assassinated. Mussolini was furious, felt threatened because of the South Tyrol, recently gained by Italy — it used to belong to Austria. Mussolini sent troops to the Italian–Austrian border to oppose the Nazis. Hitler immediately declared in the Reichstag that he has no intention whatsoever to take over Austria — "

"The liar — "

"Well, it is the fault of the British. In the Versailles Treaty of 1918, the British and French literally ruined Germany, causing tremendous inflation, unemployment, hunger, and national humiliation. On top of that came the Spanish 'flu — "

"You are right. Actually, the British lost the Great War in 1917. Of the three allies, the Russians unilaterally quit the war in 1917 and made separate peace with the Germans in the Brest–Litovsk Treaty. The French were totally demoralized and lost 600,000 young men, the flower of the nation. They were on the verge of mutiny. The British were left alone, suffered tremendous losses in East and West, the Ottoman Djemal Pasha and the German general, Kress von Kressenstein, defeated them in Palestine and threatened Suez. And the Germans ruled the seas with their submarines — "

"And what saved them was that the USA entered the war in 1917. That is why the Germans felt that the hard-earned victory was snatched from them, that they were betrayed, and, in Hitler's words, they were 'stabbed in the back' — "

"And Hitler blamed the Jews for it — "

"But what worries me most is the swift acceleration of events — "

"What made him such a rabid anti-Semite?"

"Nobody knows, maybe because at least six leaders of the communist uprising in Germany in 1919, including Rosa Luxemburg and Karl Liebknecht, were Jewish — "

"That may have contributed to it."

Neither Helene nor Edith entered the discussion but both of them felt shaken.

"No," said Helene. "They exaggerate; they are pessimists . . ."

"Maybe," said Edith.

After lunch, Edith felt quite energetic, probably because of Professor Grosser's "Hmm." For some time, she had planned to crisscross the fascinating city and get herself acquainted with some of its major architectural structures. The best way to do it was by walking, and, here and there, taking streetcars. She did not want to enter the buildings and museums this time. There would be sufficient opportunity for that later. Now she just wished to gain an overall impression of the city. The Domoj restaurant was close to the university, the Carolinum. The school was built by Charles IV in 1384 and was one of Europe's oldest universities. The language of teaching, of course, was Latin, until 1784, when, to satisfy the German majority of Prague, it was replaced by German; one hundred years later, it became bilingual: German and Czech. Unfortunately, there was a growing dispute between the two factions.

The charming Theatre or Opera of Estates was part of the university. In this magnificent theatre, Mozart personally conducted the world premiere of *Don Giovanni*. Mozart loved Prague; he wrote his Prague Symphony no. 8 to honour the city. The Czechs love music. "Every Czech is a musician," they used to say, and the city was full of music.

Prague was a large, ancient city, studded with architectural marvels of diverse styles, and was divided by the Moldava (Vltava) River. It had more than one million inhabitants, more than half of them Czech, with many Germans, particularly

Silesians. The Czechs were steadily outgrowing the German population. There were more than three million Germans in the country, including the Sudetens. The population of Czechoslovakia was 13.5 million. Until the Great War (later called World War I), they were part of the Austro-Hungarian Empire under the Hapsburgs.

Proceeding north and toward the right, Edith would have reached the lively Wenceslas (Czech Vaclav) Square, already well known to her, lined on both sides with hotels, night clubs, classy restaurants, and exquisite shops. It is the favourite meeting place of the youth, particularly around the Wenceslas statue. Wenceslas is the patron saint of Bohemia. He was murdered by his brother more than one thousand years ago.

Edith walked north and to the left, wishing to reach the Old Town Square. Passing through narrow, cobblestone-covered streets, her thoughts kept running back to the cadaver of the elderly woman, lying on the grey marble block. *Did she walk these streets? What may have been her hopes, her dreams, fears, and pains?* Edith had to bite her tongue to shush her thoughts away. Yes, the narrow streets. Once she heard that the medieval streets were purposely built narrow, so that one soldier by himself could block it with a single spear.

Unexpectedly, Edith found herself in the middle of the Old Town Square and she was stunned by the huge size of it. The Gothic mansions, palaces, innumerable churches, towers, and the statue of the martyred Jan Hus dominated the square. There was the Old City Hall with the spectacular town clock, a large instrument combining an astronomical, calendar, and time clock with the image of the twelve apostles; it was built in 1410, repaired several times, and was still working. The astonishing, but out-of-style, art nouveau Municipal House contained the huge Smetana Hall with its unique glass dome, where President Masaryk proclaimed the Czechoslovak Republic in 1918. It also housed the largest concert hall of the city, and shops, conference halls, nightclubs, restaurants, and assorted commercial businesses were there. Still on the square was the elegant Kinsky Palace, the twin-towered cathedral, the Renaissance Winter Palace, then some towers that served as jails at one time, and the Lopkowitz Palace, where the Czech crown jewels were kept in the past.

Farther north, at the elbow of the Moldava River, was Josefov, the ancient Jewish town with the ancient Jewish cemetery and with the legendary clay remains of the "Golem," built by Rebbe Low in the Middle Ages "to defend the Jews against a pending pogrom." Edith planned to spend more time there on another occasion. Instead, she turned left, toward the river, where she found Rudolfium, a neo-Renaissance building with a beautiful facade, raised for a concert hall and art centre with the patronage of Crown Prince Rudolf of Hapsburg. Currently, it accommodated the Czechoslovak Parliament.

Just three or four streets down was the sombre Clementinum (Czechs spell it "Klementinum"), a one-time Dominican Monastery, then Jesuit college, which became the city library and depository of national documents. It also housed the meteorological observatory and formed part of the university.

From the river side of the Clementinum, the Charles bridge suddenly appeared, like a spellbinding jewel, like the ornamental bracelet of a fine lady. Again, it was Charles IV, the builder king, who started its construction in 1357, connecting the Old Town with Prague Castle in the Lesser Town, across the Moldava River. The sixteen arches of the bridge are guarded by large Gothic towers on each end of the bridge, watching over the numerous Baroque sculptures of Prague's favourite saints. There is the bronze sculpture of Nepomuk; touching it is supposed to bring good luck. Another curiosity is the crucifixion scene with gold Hebrew letters: "Holy, Holy, the Lord of the Host," a quotation from a Hebrew prayer added as punishment for the Jewish community because of an alleged blasphemy in the seventeenth century. The bridge was damaged by a flood in the Middle Ages, but repaired time and time again. When its lanterns light up at dawn, the scenery becomes a magical fairy tale. Edith crossed the bridge, enjoying the boiling life around herself.

Edith bought some roasted chestnuts in a paper twist from a street vendor to munch on and continued her excursion.

Some two or three streetcar stops later, the enormous

Prague Castle complex came into view, consisting of many structures erected at different times, displaying architectural styles from Romanesque, Gothic, Renaissance, and Baroque. The first structure was built by Prince Borivoy in the year 870: the Church of Our Lady, the Basilica of St. Vitus, followed finally by the Royal Palace. As with the sequences of styles, the chronology of historic events also left their marks on the constructions, as they recalled the devastation of Prague's fire in 1541, the Swedish occupation in 1648, the Thirty Year War, floods, and epidemics. Maria Theresa rebuilt the Royal Palace where the emperor's lodging and offices were housed and where the Bohemian crown jewels had been relocated. Currently, it is the home of the eighty-four-year-old Czechoslovak president, Tomas Masaryk. The Prague Castle complex has several elaborate gardens. Much of Prague Castle is open to the public.

Exhausted, Edith did not take advantage of that privilege but sat down on a bench in one of the gardens. The flowers were gone by now, and bare bush branches offered some red berries for the birds. Yellow, orange, red, and brown crumbly leaves whooshed in a breeze announcing the coming of late autumn. A cold sigh made Edith shiver. Time to go home.

Weary, on her way home through the Legion Bridge, Edith could see from the streetcar window the National Theatre, home and essence of Bohemian culture from 1883, with stages for opera, drama, ballet, and concerts. It is the one-time home of the Prague Philharmonic Orchestra, where conductor Vaclav Talich ruled and where past giants of music such as Grieg, Rachmaninov, Mahler, and many others acted as guest conductors. The National Theatre was well known to Edith by now.

She changed streetcars and arrived at home. Her landlady, Jolana Karel, was up and waiting for Edith. "Come, have some hot tea and toast. I bought some Slovak smoked cheese, Oshtepka, just for you."

CHAPTER THREE

"Quick, quick, hurry! There is a long-distance call from Zilina, your mother . . ." Jolana Karel burst into Edith's room.

Drunk from sleep—Edith had studied till 3:20 in the morning—she jumped out of bed, heart pounding. Wearing a nightgown only, she entered Jolana's bedroom, where the telephone was located. Yes, it was Aranka on the line.

"Everything is all right, sweetheart. I just wanted to hear your voice, my dearest daughter, *moya dusha*. How are you? Are you well?"

Jolana stood beside Edith, holding Edith's housecoat and slippers.

"Yes, Mom, all is well."

"Are you eating enough?"

"Oh, yes—there is a small restaurant near the university."

"I am constantly worried about you."

"No need. Any news at home?"

"Well, Uncle Bela's little daughter, Vera, four years old now, has a swollen jaw. It is sarcoma."

"Sarcoma? It is deadly, particularly for children."

"I know it. Bela is taking her to a specialist in Budapest. Uncle Zsiga arranged it; they will stay in Zsiga's garden house."

"How is Father?"

"He is well . . . impatient with the boys, with me too . . ."

"And the boys?"

"Laci stopped school. He is learning mechanics now at Siemens. Zoli still goes to school. How are you doing with your studies?"

"I did well on the anatomy demonstration—"

"I knew you would. Please write to us."

"Yes, of course – goodbye."

"All is right?"

"Yes, Jolana, yes."

"You should not stay up so late," said Jolana disapprovingly.

Edith thought about Uncle Bela, one of the younger uncles, the least successful among the Kohns, and who had had bad luck all his life. He had been barely seventeen when he was called to arms for the Austro-Hungarian army. All of the Kohns, with the exception of Joseph, and all of the Bocks were drafted to fight in the Great War. Off to the Russian front, Bela was promptly captured and taken to Siberia as a prisoner of war. He spent more than five years in Siberia and did not come home till the early twenties. Bela got married, but every business he started went sour. He was also lazy, having gotten used to doing nothing in Siberia except gambling. And now, his little daughter had developed sarcoma.

Yes, Edith studied till the late hours. She had a near-photographic memory, but the material seemed to be endless. She knew that she was burning the candle at both ends, as the saying goes, but she was not willing to sacrifice her new-found social life, nor her medical studies. She sat with Helene and their friends in the coffee houses, chatting about art and politics; or went to concerts at cheap student prices; or movies . . . there was so much to see! And she always was an avid reader. She recently bought Thomas Mann's *Magic Mountain*, but she had not read it yet. With her medical studies and social life, she barely managed to read but a few pages. She enjoyed the Cori lecture, thought him to be a genius. Cori was an energetic character with an entirely different style from Grosser's.

"Every energy derives from the sun," Cori said, while he walked to the large blackboard with chalk in his hand. He drew a circle with rays around it. "This is the sun," he said. Then he drew a little "man" with four lines carrying a sort of briefcase, walking toward a "building" that he sketched. On that, he scribbled the word "bank."

"That is physiology. We live a busy life, costing energy, and we have no time to waste. Who has time? The trees have time."

He drafted a sort of tree behind the little guy. "The trees have time. The leaves spread out and chemically encapsulate the sun's energy, the process called photosynthesis. Our busy guy eats the leaves, the locked-in energy will be released, and our man has fuel to use. Life, as we know it, is a self-perpetuating process assured by the photosynthesis of carbon, hydrogen, and oxygen, yielding carbohydrates, including ribosin, which then produces DNA and RNA. This is physiology, the rest are details, and my assistant will teach you the particulars."

Simple, charismatic, yet a never-heard-of summary. One never can forget the essence that he had outlined with a few words. He had laid open the principle of life itself.

Back at home, Edith took a shower and, while she dried herself, she heard the radio playing somewhere in the neighbourhood the new Cole Porter song, "I Get a Kick Out of You." Once those songs were picked up, you could hear them all the time.

Off to the university. She was busy non-stop, till late in the afternoon on this cold, rainy November day. She could hardly believe the news that the Rector, Karel Domin, on the Czech side of the university, had encouraged the Czech students to fetch the ancient insignia back from the German section, using violence, if need be. This back-and-forth argument about Charles IV's insignia or seal had gone on at least for two years, and thousands of Czech students had demonstrated in front of the German University the other day.

Today, Rector Otto Grosser had transferred the troublesome seal to the Czech University. Grosser did that to prevent violence and any further splitting between the Czech and German universities. *This won't be viewed kindly either by Hitler or by the Silesian Germans* thought Edith. The overheard discussion at Domoj the other day flashed through her mind. *Are we really heading to a national catastrophe?* she asked herself. *No — the British-French Treaty can be relied on.*

Helene was supposed to drop in in the afternoon. Shoeless, stretched out on her bed, Edith browsed through the paper and was almost finished when a knock on her door roused her. Helene came in.

"What did you think of the Cori lecture?" Edith asked.

"A genius," replied Helene.

"You seem to have a sour face," noted Edith.

"No, not really. Well, something is bothering me. I can't get off my mind the social and professional discrimination against us women. What we have to put up with! Did you hear the other day Professor Grosser's derogatory words about us female medical students? And this is in the supposedly democratic Czechoslovakia. 'Women should stay home and look after husband and children.' The fabricated notion that women's brains are not adapted for science. What about Mme. Curie? The female brain is not suited to grasp mathematics? Despite the ancient Hypatia and the legion of woman mathematicians since then?"

"Well, that's old hat. What is really bothering you?"

Helene hesitated. "Well, if you want to know, this is my first day of my moon time."

"There is some good in it."

"Good? What?" asked Helene.

"That your sins did not start germinating."

Helene became quiet.

Edith said, "I saw you the other day making big eyes at Marcus Pavel."

"You devil. Don't worry, Edith, I know my cycle. And you?"

"I am a saint and a virgin."

"Hah!"

"Should we go to the movies?"

"Well, Czech movies need to grow up. German movies are full of propaganda these days, like the Russian movies, with the exception of Sergei Eisenstein. That leaves us the American and French movies—sometimes the British, particularly if they are produced by foreigners, like Alexander Korda."

"Let's look at the paper. There is a Czech comedy with Jan Sebor; then a Marlene Dietrich film, *The Scarlet Empress*—this is her American film; then *It Happened One Night*, with Clark Gable and Claudette Colbert; then *The Gay Divorcee* with Fred Astaire and Ginger Rogers—an Academy Award winner; then another Claudette Colbert movie, *Cleopatra*."

"Where does it play?"

"Kino Lucerna. You know, that fancy old place."

"Let us go to that one."

"We should have chosen the Clark Gable movie," said Helene on their way out.

"It was not bad, and it was quite showy." Edith's faint praise sounded more like an agreement with her girlfriend.

Later during the week, Edith ran into Klara Novak, the philosophy major, on the street. On seeing Edith, Klara exclaimed: "Just the person I wished to see!" Klara did not lunch often at the Domoj.

Edith respected the mind of this young woman. Whenever they met, and whatever topic happened to come in focus, Klara remained calm and passed a discerned, circumspect opinion; her thoughts always ran deep. She was quite different than the rest of the students. She was good-looking and had natural, beautiful skin that required little, if any, makeup; and long, dark-brown hair falling onto her shoulders. Klara always dressed in quality clothing, with not much emphasis on current fashion. She spoke flawless Czech and German — both were her mother tongues — and managed a good conversation in French and English. She had always been a good student and excelled in mathematics. Since childhood, she was a fervid reader and a lover of music. She played the piano but just for herself.

"I am an easy target to find," laughed Edith.

"Well, just the person I wished to find. I know that you are terribly busy. I hear that some of your professors would like to see all girls married, in the kitchen, and pregnant. So, you must work extra hard, I guess. I see you've lost some weight since I saw you last.

"But what I want to tell you, some of us have a little literary circle . . . no, not like Berta Fanta's famous literary circle, of course, but we have some very bright people with a good sense of humour amongst us. You would enjoy it. We meet once every two weeks . . . I mean, at my place . . ."

"Why, I am honoured and pleased. Once in two weeks is still manageable. But tell me about Berta Fanta. I keep hearing her name. I know she lived in Prague but very little else."

"Berta Fanta . . . Berta Fanta," Klara closed her eyes as if in deep thought. "Berta Fanta was a brilliant woman from a rich Jewish-Czech family who studied philosophy at the German University of Prague, travelled, lived an enriching cultural life around the turn of the century. She had boundless energy, a real doer. She transformed her house into a magnet of cultured people, where every Tuesday outstanding minds met and mingled: writers, scientists, poets, composers, philosophers . . . male and female. More than anybody else, she made Prague the cultural centre for local and for itinerant eager participants, like Sofia Kovalevskaya, the superb Russian mathematician, who, being female, was not even allowed to attend university in her native country but became Professor Ordinarius in Sweden; and like Albert Einstein, and Thomas Mann, and Karel Capec, who in his futuristic novels invented the concept of 'robot'; like the lawyer Franz Kafka, who changed modern literature; like Jaroslav Hilbert, playwright; Franz Werfel; the mystical philosopher Martin Buber; and many others. Berta Fanta died of a heart attack sixteen years ago, just when she was in the process of immigrating to Palestine. If you want, I can show you Berta's house. Now, we are not competing with Berta Fanta — we are lightweights, doing it just for fun. Will you come? The next meeting is day after tomorrow at my place."

"I shall certainly be there," said Edith.

"Here is my address." Klara handed Edith a printed card bearing her name and address.

Edith spent the entire next day at home in the company of her Sobotta anatomy atlas. She had a cold chicken sandwich for lunch with strong black coffee while she scrutinized the drawings and fine print, observing nerves, vessels, and tendons traversing each other. By the afternoon she was cross-eyed from reading the small print over the illustrations. She closed her eyes from exhaustion, thought of the splash and swoosh of the Vah River bubbling forth over scattered rocks; she could even smell the aroma of pine trees, wild mushrooms, and yellow crocuses . . . with the book in her hand, she fell into a deep sleep.

She woke suddenly in mid-afternoon. She was afraid that she would be late, but in fact she had plenty of time. At 7:00 p.m., the official "get acquainted party" of the university was to be held in the dining room and hall of one of the Wenceslas Square hotels.

Edith had a shower and put on her makeup—red lipstick and faint, dark eye shadow. She put on her black evening gown with a V-shaped décolleté, showing her figure favourably, and with a loose-fitting skirt suited for dancing, the hem of which reached just beneath her knees. She twisted a long bijou pearl chain around her neck, pulled on dark silk stockings held up by a corselette, and stepped into a pair of dancing shoes. She looked in the mirror and was satisfied with her "look." Adjusting her hair, administering a tiny splash of Mitsouko Guerlain, which she had learned from Aunt Sarah in Budapest (never used it at the university), and she was ready to go.

In the dining room, on her right sat Markus Povel with Helene, and on Edith's left Alexej Pavel, a second-year engineering student with cropped hair and red acne on his chin. He was from the industrial city of Brun. Alexej was somewhat awkward, rigid. Edith wondered why Alexej had chosen to come to Prague for his studies, when in Brun there was Masaryk University and the famous Institute of Technology, not to mention the huge Skoda works. She soon learned that Alexej was a devoted gymnast, and the national team's home was in Prague.

The orchestra was playing soft salon music during dinner, and Edith observed that several boys were swarming around the officially appointed chaperons, making them drink more and more wine, toasting the university, the nation, Masaryk, Beneš, and whatever else came to mind.

Helene, seated in midst of medical students, began to imitate Professor Grosser. She combed her hair onto her forehead, fished out a pair of black-framed glasses from her handbag and, mimicking Grosser's voice and mannerisms, she said: "See, gentlemen and, alas! ladies, without anatomy you cannot even have a good time. Therefore, I say to you in Latin, a language I speak fluently, *gaudeamus igitur*, have a good time!"

A vigorous, hearty laughter followed, an all began to sing the well-known students' song, raising their glasses.

The dinner was brief, and soon the orchestra switched to foxtrot, then more foxtrot, tango, waltz, and foxtrot again. Edith passed from one dance partner to another. Finally, she had to rest. She noticed a tall, very good-looking student with dark hair and blue eyes, sitting by himself, watching the dancers. With a slight perspiration filming her brow, she sat herself beside him.

"You don't like to dance?"

"Oh, yes, but sometimes I just like to watch the dancers for a while."

"I am Edith Bock, first-year medical student. And you?"

"My name is Jan Miroslav; I am a third-year musicologist."

"Then you must play an instrument."

"Yes, I play the violin . . . but my love is really the viola."

"Oh, viola!" sighed Edith. "There is nothing more appealing for the heart than the rich, mellow, and masculine sound of the viola — but viola solos are relatively rare."

"To a degree only. But there are plenty of them, if you look."

Edith pondered. "I always thought of viola pieces as sugar."

"Sugar? Why?"

"Well, because you need sugar in everything you bake, but concentrated sugar is another matter."

Jan laughed heartily at the unexpected explanation. "Do you have any favourite viola pieces?"

Edith thought. "I know when I became prejudiced against the violin. It was when my brother was practising . . . but viola pieces . . . a difficult question . . . favourite . . . maybe Paganini's *Quartet*, recitativo . . ."

Jan laughed. "I did not know that in first-year medical school they taught Paganini . . . let's dance."

Jan turned out to be an excellent dancer. And they exchanged telephone numbers. And a light kiss on the cheek.

Chapter Four

Searching for Klara's home, Edith was frustrated; there was no apartment number marked on the printed card, and the house number was not typical of a student residence but featured a very large, luxurious villa. With much hesitation, Edith rang the bell, and a uniformed servant opened the door. Hesitantly, she inquired: "I am looking for a Miss Klara Novak."

"Please, enter. Miss Novak will be here in a minute." She was ushered to a nearby room filled with leather-covered seats, *fauteuils* (armchairs), oriental carpets, Louis IV furniture, old Baroque paintings, bookcases, porcelain figurines, and a small writing desk with real feather pen and ink horn. The room smelled of lavender and old wealth. The servant took Edith's coat.

A cheerful Klara soon walked in, hugged Edith. "You are a touch too early but just as well. The participants will arrive shortly and they like to chat a bit before the meeting starts."

Klara took Edith to another, very large room, well lit by a crystal chandelier and filled with rows of comfortable leather seats, a small table standing in front of them. On the table were a lamp and some papers. "Did you have any difficulty finding the place?"

"Well," said Edith, "frankly, I was expecting a student's nest."

"It all belongs to my parents. My father is a lawyer, a city councillor, and he comes from an old, rich family. I am just a guest here." She laughed.

Some commotion arose outside, and two men and a woman arrived, talking, joking as they entered the room. More raucous voices, and still others came. "Hey, Klara!" Hugs and kisses. Then more people arrived, and in no time the room was full, with men and women engaged in jabbering . . . as old acquaintances do.

"Come to order, friends," announced Klara two or three times in a penetrating voice. The prattle waved up and down, then slowly subsided. "I have the privilege to introduce our newest member, Edith Bock from Zilina, a first-year medical student. Be gentle with her. Currently she is involved in the mysteries of anatomy, and, while she is very young, you will enjoy her original thinking."

The little crowd burst into applause. Klara made Edith stand up. Edith blushed.

"*Magnifique!* A young medical student. We need a new mind like that!" a young man said in French. Then, switching to a heavily French-accented German, continued, "We are honored to have Mademoiselle Edith Bock in our small circle." He was Maurice, a young diplomat from the French Embassy, his first posting.

Klara announced that the results of this year's Nobel Prize of Literature were out, and the winner was Luigi Pirandello. "As the youngest member of our circle, Edith, you may wish to say a few words about that."

Edith blushed again. "Unfortunately, I do not know much about Pirandello. I read just for fun. I have seen only one of Pirandello's plays, *Six Characters in Search of an Author*, and that was an amateur performance. I must confess I did not like it. I understood that he was reaching out for something new—something different from everyday reality—but his intention does not justify his confusion.

"But I wish to take a quick look at those who were nominated for Nobel Prize this year and were turned down, like Eugene O'Neill, a brilliant playwright, and, above all, Roger Martin du Gard, my long-time favourite. The committee that awards the Nobel Prize consists of just human beings, not immune to personal and national interests and unspoken political issues. This explains why authors like Mark Twain, Leo Tolstoy, Marcel Proust, Anton Chekhov, and others like them were never awarded the Nobel Prize. Can it be that we overestimate the prize itself?"

The group burst out in applause again, making Edith's face turn red once more.

A fascinating discussion followed. Next day, a bouquet of flowers arrived at Edith's home with an ornate embassy card: "Thank you for your insightful remarks yesterday. Roger Martin du Gard happens to be my favourite, too, particularly his *Jean Barois*. Hope to see you at the next gathering. With my respect: Maurice." Edith was quite impressed.

She concentrated on her anatomy studies. No time for anything else, except a rendezvous with Jan, who had called her immediately after the university party.

More lectures followed, and lunches at the Domoj. No surprise — as usual, the same students obsessed with politics were there. Helene and Edith purposely sat at the next table, as a silent audience.

"Hitler is a genius . . . an evil genius," the girls heard one of them saying. "Look at what he has done to the German economy."

"Indeed, it is remarkable."

"When he came into power, all of Germany was a mess, just as the British wanted it. The Germans were bankrupt; they could not pay the reparation laid down in the Versailles Treaty, so the French took over the Saar industrial area, and there was inflation . . . unemployment . . . the country was on verge of revolution."

"The German mark was not worth the paper it was printed on."

"The Americans and the British had their currency backed up with gold; they ran on the gold standard. Hitler printed new Reichsmarks and backed them up by the Brown Shirts, the SA."

"But they were worthless on the international market!"

"Worthless? Maybe. But Hitler did not care about international recognition. He set the prices, the salaries for the workers, the price of bread, of fuel, the rents, and everything else within Germany. The internal economy was guaranteed by the bayonets of the SA and SS — dare to oppose them. The concentration camp Ravensbrück was awaiting them.

"The Germans had a monotonous diet in those days; zero money was spent on fancy food or imported goods."

"Except for the leadership of the party."

"That is understood."

"At any rate, there was no unemployment, and women, too, were encouraged to work in the factories."

"But Hitler wanted women to get pregnant — "

"Yes, and paid generous monetary compensation and gave maternity leaves."

"Yes, and the workers thrived."

"Hitler invented other incentives, too, like showy military parades — "

" — and promised that every family would own a very reasonably priced car, the Volkswagen — "

"But Hitler imitated Mussolini all the way. It was Mussolini who introduced the fascist greeting with the raised arm, an old Roman salutation, and it was Mussolini who pioneered the fascist youth movement, the '*Balillas*,' what Hitler called 'Hitler *Jugend*.' He even copied Mussolini's 'Strength through Joy' movement — "

"Maybe so, but it was Hitler who made it popular . . ."

Helene and Edith were amazed at what they heard.

"Yes, he offered a program he called '*Kraft durch Freude*' — the 'Strength through Joy.' Luxury liners were confiscated and factory workers were taken for pleasure cruises with their families."

"No wonder the nation became Hitler's admirer."

"And the confiscated wealth of the Jews was used to cover the U.S. dollar needs for absolutely necessary goods."

"What made him so bold?"

"Simple, it was the sheer recognition that no matter what, neither the East nor the West would enter a new war. Being so much afraid of a new military conflict, they would do anything to avoid it."

"And Hitler knew it."The overheard discussion dampened the mood of the two girls; they knew by then that these students were no fools. But the daily circumstances were still good in Czechoslovakia, and, willy-nilly, life had to go on. Yet, their views on the reliability of Eastern and Western treaties became less firm than they were before.

Edith and Jan met at the espresso bar at Wenceslas Square, the one Edith liked to visit. Jan had just come from the Conservatorium and carried his violin in its case. They had seen each other four times since the university party: twice, just chatting in the espresso bar; once at a concert (Bach's *Brandenburg Concerto* no. 2 in F Major; Schubert's *La Solitude*; Smetana's *The Secret*); and once when Jan took her out for dinner. The more conversation they had, the stronger their bond, and both of them felt a budding love emerging.

"Give up medicine. You can play piano a bit, and I know a magnificent piano teacher and composer here in Prague, Ilona Stepanova-Kurzova, who will make you a success in no time. Then we can play piano and viola together." They both laughed. Anatomy and violin — a strange combination.

"I would like to hear you play the viola."

"It can be arranged."

"How?"

"Either in the Conservatorium or in my modest little apartment."

"You mean in your love nest."

"Why not?" And they laughed again.

Soon, Edith found herself in Jan's apartment. It was indeed modest, and looked like a veritable bachelor flat. Music sheets scattered beside the unwashed breakfast dishes, an unmade bed, some amateurish pictures hanging crooked on the wall, a plant dying for water, some worn shirts in a corner.

"Feel at home and relax."

Edith was anything but relaxed. Jan lifted with careful fingers from the cabinet a viola case, and, lifting out the flannel-covered viola, caressed the shiny instrument.

"You make me jealous," mumbled Edith.

Jan put the viola to his left shoulder, tested the sound. Then he started to play. It was a never-heard-of strange melody, not very appealing.

"Do you know this piece?"

"No. Never heard it."

"It was written in the eighteenth century by Princess Anna Amalia of Prussia, sister of Frederick II." Jan started to play again, just a fragment. The deep, glowing tone filled the room but it was also unfamiliar to Edith. "A little-known creation of Carl Stamitz, a real virtuoso. It sounds even better when played on viola d'amore." Jan then played a short part of Vivaldi's violin concerto.

Soon the viola was back in its case, and the two of them sat side by side. Jan hesitantly put his hand on Edith's shoulder. They turned face to face, and Jan gently kissed Edith's lips. That is how the two of them became lovers.

CHAPTER FIVE

Well, it happened. Edith was in shock. What a disaster! She should have been more careful. Almost failed her midterm physiology examination—because she had been carried away with her extensive social life and all the other distractions. Right there and then, she decided that she must cut her frivolous activities to a minimum.

Oh, no, but not Jan! Jan became her passion, her love, the object of her devotion. Their trysts, now mainly in Jan's little apartment, gave her a hitherto unknown quivering sensation; their intimacy reached a throbbing zest. She would always keep up with Klara's bimonthly meetings, too, and, of course, in the slimmed-down time, the Domoj lunches with her good friend Helene. But all her other diversions, concerts included, must go! And the tennis matches with Helene, who beat her regularly, as well.

The monotony of her daily studies from morning to midnight made time vanish unnoticed. Only her meetings with Jan broke her rigorous schedule. One evening, the room was lit only by the feeble glint of a single bulb sneaking in from the open kitchen door and by two glowing cigarettes. Jan, totally nude, got up and opened his precious cabinet. Too dark to see, Edith guessed that he was reaching for his viola. But instead of a viola, Edith realized, only when Jan started to play, that he had lifted out a clarinet. The opening glissando of *Rhapsody in Blue*, like a precious gift, filled the tiny room with its challenging tone. Double surprise for Edith. Clarinet? And classical jazz?

Jan laughed. "I love clarinet. Besides, I sometimes play in a jazz orchestra in a nightclub when money runs short."

"Gershwin worked it out on a train ride, you know. You can even hear the rhythmic noises of the train composed into it in some parts," observed Edith.

"And the din of New York City as well," noted Jan.

"Did you have anybody else in your life before me?" asked Edith.

"Yes . . . I had an affair with a girl, Vera, from the nightclub where I played in the jazz orchestra. But it is all over and past," replied Jan.

Before they knew it, New Year's sneaked up on them unnoticed. The two of them went to a student party to celebrate. Lots of dancing, quite a lot of drinking, then the room went almost completely dark, and, in the cacophony of human clamour and musical instruments, the year 1935 was born.

"What will it bring?"

"We are in the hands of Providence."

Over lunch at the Domoj, Edith told Helene about Klara's literary circle. Helene made a funny face. "What?" asked Edith.

"Well, didn't you know?"

"Know what?"

"That Klara is a lesbian. Not that it matters much. Just so you know."

"It is new to me."

"It doesn't matter. You are not her type anyway. She goes for barmaids. She drops by at a lesbian strip club sometimes."

"How did you know that?"

"In a certain sense, Prague is a small village."

"I guess she is entitled to her choice," observed Edith.

"Just as you are to yours," said Helene meaningfully.

At the Domoj, Edith and Helene continued to pick up more and more alarming political news from an increasing number of concerned students. They all revolved around the martial German regime, now openly evolving into a perilous threat, which the unprepared British and French pretended not to notice. In 1922, the Western powers had taken over the heavily industrialized Saarland from a then dying Germany unable to pay reparations. Now, in January 1935, through Hitler's insistence, a plebiscite took place under the League of Nations' supervision, and, thanks to pre-contrived Nazi propaganda, over 90 percent of the population chose to be reunited with Germany. The triumph has been appropriately dramatized by German military troops marching into Saar, in close lines, with high-flying swastika flags, military bands playing fiery marching songs and the SA hymn: "*Die Fahne hoch, die Reihe fest geschlossen, SA marschiert —* " ("The flags fly high, the lines in tight formation, SA marching — ")

Artillery and tanks followed the marching forces, pretending that the legitimate accession was not a political agreement but a daring military victory. By then, Germany had openly overstepped the military limits laid down in the Versailles Treaty. The German factories were pouring out ammunition, weapons, artillery, submarines, and a large number of high-quality warplanes. The latter gave Czechoslovakia particular concern, for their own best defence was their air force. While the Versailles Treaty permitted Germany only up to 100,000 soldiers at any given time, the SA alone numbered 2.5 million. Obligatory conscription was re-established in the spring of 1935.

It was not that the British and French were unaware of all the preparations taking place on German soil; but their own unpreparedness, and the population's dread of a possible new military conflict, dictated Western foreign policy. It was Hitler's greatest strength that he was perfectly aware of these facts, which consequently permitted him to make outrageous demands. He constantly was testing just how far he could go. The strictly isolationist United States, deep in the Depression, was struggling with Roosevelt's New Deal.

Tentative plans to move the venue of the XI Olympic Games, Hitler's toy, joy, and pride, which had been awarded to Germany in pre-Nazi times, fell through. A planned boycott by the United States had collapsed when the head of the American Olympic Committee, Avery Brundage, was sent to Germany. There, he was received with the highest honour and was assured that Jewish athletes would have equal but separate facilities. Among other issues, Brundage was politely asked just how many Jewish members there were in the New York Athletic Club. Of course, they knew the answer: none. Brundage and his inspection team returned to New York with the opinion that the Jewish athletes in Germany "are treated fairly, and there is a Jewish-Communist effort afoot that wants to keep the United States out of the Olympics." Neither the United Kingdom nor France boycotted the Olympics.

The months passed swiftly with long and weary labour. When spring came, the fragrance of blooming lilacs swept in through Edith's open window, and she fought hard not to give in to her youthful urge to run to the nearby park and roll around in the soft grass. Time for the examination arrived before Edith knew it.

There was a single cadaver on the marble table. Edith and five other students, wearing rubber gloves and immaculate white gowns, stood in the Dissection Hall in front of Professor Otto Grosser, all of them nervous and shaky, with some demonstrators congregating in the background.

"Expose for me, Mr. Fritz Schulz, the ulnar nerve." Edith saw the Silesian boy make a cut on the right lower arm, and she immediately knew that Schulz wouldn't make it. Schulz searched the subcutaneous tissues, a bewildering array of tendons, vessels, and the wrong nerves with shaky hands. He was sweating.

"Enough; you failed," said Grosser. "Next: Mr. Pavel Jaroslav."

Schulz walked away with a grey face. "Now, Mr. Jaroslav, open up the facial artery." Jaroslav, too, made the cut in the wrong place. "Failed!" said Grosser in a raised voice. "What is the matter with this class?" he addressed the demonstrators. "They must have been sleeping all these months!"

Edith felt a knot in her stomach. "Edith Bock." Evidently Grosser recognized her. "I permit you a one-centimeter cut. Locate for me the lateral peroneal nerve." A slight murmur rose up in the midst of the demonstrators who knew the extraordinary difficulty of the task. Edith laid both palms on the cadaver's right knee, slowly moving them around, searching for the bony protuberance at the outer side, just beneath the knee. When she found it, she laid her left pointing finger on the knob, right hand reaching for the knife. She made her small cut just above the bony protuberance, the left-hand thumb and pointing finger stretching open the incision, while her right hand found the shiny metal hook. She entered the hook into the opened furrow, lifting gently the yellow nerve to be visible for Grosser.

And then something unheard-of happened: Grosser said, loud and clear: "Excellent! You passed the examination with an excellent mark. Now: This is not the examination anymore. Would you know any pathology connected with this nerve?"

"Entrapment at various levels, I guess."

Grosser turned to the remaining two students. "Maybe you all could learn from this lady." Then he turned to Edith. "Do you know anyone with such an ailment?"

"No," answered Edith.

The demonstrators remarked to Edith: "We should probably notify the archivist of the university. It has never happened before that Professor Grosser was so generous with his praise."

Edith felt slightly nauseous; her head was swimming. But she went to the Domoj to meet Helene, who had also passed the examination in another room, by another examiner. She had passed it with a "sufficient" mark but she was very happy. Helene already knew about Edith's success. The two friends spent quite a long time together, chatting.

It was late afternoon and, still in an exuberant mood, Edith decided to surprise Jan at his apartment, to tell him about her triumph. She used a touch of Mitsouko to take away the lingering smell of formaldehyde. She anticipated the joy shining on Jan's face, hearing of her success — that is, if she found him at home. She walked up the familiar stairs and the ill-lit corridor and reached for the door handle; the door was open. Suddenly Edith found herself facing a straw-blonde, braless woman wearing only panties, a cigarette dangling from her lips. For a split second, Edith thought she was on the wrong floor. But no. Then she knew. Vera. Then she saw Jan coming out from the kitchen, in underpants and open shirt. Edith stood there gaping, her mind refusing to grasp what her eyes had seen. Then she ran and ran, too shocked to cry yet.

She found a luxury hotel nearby, ran to the ladies room, locked herself in a stall, and cried and cried. She thought that she would never stop crying. After a while, she composed herself. From the hotel lobby she called Helene. "Come, come to my place immediately!" And Edith ran home as if she were being chased by demons.

Helene was holding her tight, and both of them were crying together, Helene grasping the pain without words, as only women can do. She wanted Edith to stay at her place overnight, but Edith chose the solitude of her own room.

"You have a basketful of messages from the same man, asking me to tell you to call him back. It is urgent," Jolana informed her, guessing the ongoing drama. Edith took the phone number, which was well known to her, and told Jolana that whoever calls, she was "not at home."

Without undressing, Edith threw herself on her bed and cried into her pillow until it was wet. She heard several times a silent, knowing Jolana entering her room; at one point, covering her with a blanket.

The following morning, Edith had to go to the Questura to look after official matters but soon returned home. A huge bouquet of flowers and a letter from Jan were waiting for her. The letter from Jan begged her to give him an opportunity "to explain everything."

Jolana said just one sarcastic word: "Men."

Edith chose not to answer Jan. Soon the telephone rang, and Jolana called Edith. Of course, it was Jan. He begged Edith for a chance to meet in the espresso bar; he needed to explain everything. Edith wavered but accepted.

"You see, I had a long relationship with Vera. I knew her from the nightclub where I played in the jazz orchestra. I broke off with her before we met. But Vera was crying, calling me all the time; she was hysterical and threatened to kill herself. Finally, I saw her and felt sorry for her. That is how it happened, but it is over now, I swear."

"But you kept it a secret from me. And I could see that it was more than just pity on your part. Do you want to feel pity for me, too?" Edith felt that no matter what, things would never be the same again. And regardless of how much it hurt, she was not ready to settle for less.

The study break came up, and Edith was to return home for the summer. Near to Milady Horakove, north of Lesser Town, she boarded her train to Zilina with a bag full of laundry and her Sobotta. On the train, she kept thinking of all the ups and downs of the last year, and finally tried to read *The Magic Mountain*. But the train, with crossing rails and small bridges, became a veritable orchestra for Edith with its rhythmic puffing of steam and metallic clatter of steel wheels, imitating the glissando of the *Rhapsody in Blue* . . . bringing on a new flood of tears.

CHAPTER SIX

When the rattling train pulled into the small, mustard-yellow terminal of Zilina, it was already dark. The Bock family, waiting impatiently, burst into hoot and holler as the train came to a shuddering halt. Edith, leaning out the window, was waving. The boys climbed onto the still-moving car to grab Edith's luggage and coat. With hugs and kisses, they ushered her to Hugo's car, simultaneously raising too many questions to answer as they neared the family home. All lights were on, Aranka running to the kitchen to check on the food. Father, with unpractised fingers, opened a champagne bottle, sixteen-year-old Laci got a few drops of it, Zolo demanded to taste it at least, and in the confusion everyone got his or her way.

Mother brought the steaming mushroom soup to the dining room (*Learn, Domoj,* thought Edith), and everyone talked at the same time, nobody grasping what the other was saying in the happy cacophony. It took a while for the family to settle down. Aranka prepared all the dishes Edith liked, and food was left over for many days. After supper, Mother straightened her apron and began to clear the table, but Edith would not let her. The boys finished the job, although, with one ear inside the dining room, they were dying to hear every word said.

Father lit a cigar and Edith lit a cigarette. "Are you smoking?" asked a surprised Aranka disapprovingly. Then, in a quieter tone, Edith gave an account of everything. She talked about Jolana — "bless her heart," sighed Aranka — then she reflected on the Domoj, on Helene, on the examinations, and spoke at length of Prague in general. Not a word about Jan, of course. Hugo commented on the growing anti-Semitism in Slovakia, about his fear of the spreading Nazism; Edith tried to mitigate his concerns, despite her own apprehension.

Exhausted by joy, the family was slowly fading. Happiness is tiring. First the boys bowed out, then all of them were overtaken by languor, assisted by the champagne.

Sleeping in her own bed once again was a great pleasure for Edith. Stretching her limbs on the snow-white, freshly laundered bed linen, like a lazy cat, she enjoyed how her bed hugged her exhausted body. With the light out now, the deep silence of the small town around her, she almost missed the night-and-day rumble of the metropolis she had gotten used to. She vaguely heard a dog barking in the distance before she fell into a deep sleep. She awakened briefly at the first blush of daylight, as she used to in Prague, but then she gave in to the cuddling comfort of her bed, and slumbered on.

She awakened to the soft clatter of dishes, the household noises, and the tempting aroma of the brewing morning coffee seeping through the closed bedroom door. She put on her housecoat and slippers and found Aranka preparing breakfast in the kitchen. Finally, a chance for some private women's talk. "How is Father?"

"Somewhat better. He is more confident about our future but I still worry about him. The business is very good, keeps him busy, and that helps."

"And the boys?"

"They spend a lot of time at the Sokol, a Jewish sport facility run by the Zionists. Imagine, your thirteen-year-old cousin, Zsuzsa, wants to immigrate to Palestine."

After breakfast, Edith visited some of the family. One of the oldest Kohn boys, Sandor, a very rich man, owned a big house where the grandparents lived in one of the apartments. Grandma Franciska spoke German only, for she came from Alsace–Lothringen. Most of the Kohns spoke three languages: German, Slovak, and the older ones also Hungarian, for Slovakia used to belong to Hungary till the end of the Great War. Edith, too, spoke Hungarian, Slovak, Czech, German, and a bit of French as well, which had been an obligatory course in her gymnasium (a secondary school that prepares students for entrance to university), besides Latin.

Sandor had finished gymnasium but did not study any further. He was a self-made man, a devoted reader, and an excellent businessman. He also owned a mirror factory. Sandor used to give a gold coin to every niece and nephew for their birthday. When Edith met him visiting Grandma, Sandor pulled Edith aside and slipped into her hand a small deerskin purse filled with fifteen Napoleon gold coins. Edith did not want to take it, but Sandor insisted.

By now, most of Zilina knew that Edith was back at home. In a small town, news scurries swiftly. Floods of telephone calls came to the house. Edith wished to pay a surprise visit to her father's store at the city square. The square is lined all around with early eighteenth-century, two- or three-storey houses, each with an arcade in the front, covering and protecting a passageway for the public. The ground floor of these buildings housed varieties of stores, restaurants, coffee houses, pubs, and ice cream parlours. The cobblestone-covered plaza offered occasional fruit stalls and an open-wagon farmer's market with bored horses standing in harness, tossing their big heads up and down, vexed by insistent flies that made their shiny, brown skins quiver while their stringy tails swished them away.

The square served as an informal meeting place where Edith ran into friends, bygone schoolmates, earlier teachers, and yesterday's boyfriends. She was loved, envied, and gossiped about by so many people. She met Uncle Bela walking with his wife, Honora, and their six-year-old daughter, Judith. The family were still mourning the recent passing of their little daughter Vera.

Laci and Zolo decided to take a whole day's excursion with Edith in the area of the Lower Tatra Mountain. They wore boots and backpacks filled with swimsuits, towels, and sandwiches, and carried alpenstocks. Early morning fog was still floating around as they departed at daybreak. They took a brief train ride to Liptovsky Mikulas, a resort town, also at the shore of the Vah River. Soon the scenery became more rustic. From there, they walked north, singing old, silly songs they remembered from childhood, and their steps became lighter.

In the background, grey, rocky mountains soared toward the sky, the peaks of some covered by snow, others draped in cottony white clouds. They passed green, dewy fields covered in multicoloured wildflowers — forget-me-nots, crocuses, yellow buttercups — and wild blueberries, unobtrusively engaged in a slow, silent territorial combat with one another. Then came muddy trails with moss-covered rocks and coniferous evergreen forests.

Soon they found a crystal-clear lake, then some ancient caves. They ran out of songs. Climbing the terrain, breathing became punctuated with gasping breaths, and they gratefully used their alpenstocks. Suddenly, they found themselves in an emerald-green clearing, where they surprised a group of some thirty or so deer, standing motionless, attentive, with bulging eyes, ears turned forward; then, without a noticeable signal, they broke into a fast run, disappearing between the trees.

In this idyllic spot, the three of them settled on the shore of a small rivulet. They ate their sandwiches and drank virgin clean water, right from the racing brook, which was lined with waxy yellow flowers. The brook was too cold for swimming. They were looking for edelweiss but could not find any. The pristine cool air permeated their lungs, and, used to the city atmosphere, it was a rare, refreshing experience. Edith pointed out a pair of eagles circling the sky with majestic, motionless, outstretched wings. Time to return home. By the time they reached Liptovsky Mikulas, the crickets, wearing their formal black attire, were tuning their instruments for their night's concert.

"You had a long-distance call. From Bratislava — Helene called."

It was too late to call her back; it must wait till the morning.

For some time, Edith had intended to pay a visit to Uncle Zsiga (sobriquet for Sigmund) and his family in Budapest and to look around for a possible two- or three-month internship in that busy city. A new regulation by the university permitted such internships to be completed during the summer months from the second year on, in order to shorten the overall training time. Edith discussed it with her parents.

The decision made, Hugo informed the family that he was closing the shop for a week and would drive Aranka and Edith to Budapest. The boys would stay with Sandor, there not being enough room in the car. If Edith's business required it, she could return later by train. Edith was delighted. Not the boys, though, for Sandor was a disciplinarian.

In the morning, Edith called Helene and told her about the family plan. Helene persuaded her to break up the return trip at Bratislava and stay with her for a few days. A wonderful idea!

Within a short time, the travellers were ready to depart. The store and the house were locked up, the keys and the reluctant boys were handed over to Sandor, the car was checked by the mechanic, and at daybreak they were on their way to Budapest. It was a long trip, considering the poor quality of the road and the always unpleasant border crossing between Czechoslovakia and Hungary.

The relation between the Slovaks and the Hungarians was hostile, to say the least. It is remarkable because both were mainly agricultural countries, both ruled by the leftover feudalistic regimes. Unlike the Czechs, both Slovaks and Hungarians were devoted Roman Catholics and, until the end of the Great War, both shared poverty as well. But the Austrians snubbed the Hungarians, and the Hungarians scorned the Slovaks. Slovakia was ruled by the Hungarians, and even after the Great War, Hungarians, particularly the Hungarian aristocracy, owned much of Slovakia and used the Slovaks as cheap labour. The Hungarians hated the Slovaks, for they broke away from "Greater Hungary."

Consequently, they made life difficult for one another, wherever they could. One such opportunity was the border crossing, where travellers, regardless of their nationality, were treated by both sides as enemy spies or criminals. The border crossing endured for hours, and was made as unpleasant an experience as possible.

No wonder the family was exhausted upon their late evening arrival. Zsiga's mother tongue was German; he also spoke good Slovak but only a very poor Hungarian that he had picked up upon marrying Sarah in Budapest in 1917. The Bock family, except for the boys, spoke good Hungarian. Zsiga, isolated from his parents and siblings in Hungary, was delighted when a rare opportunity arose to see them. Zsiga's wife, Sarah, prepared an outstanding dinner for the family, and the Bocks stayed with them in Zsiga's summer cottage in Buda located in a beautiful rose garden, with fruit trees and a sparkling water fountain. Zsiga's children, fifteen-year-old Marta and twelve-year-old Erwin (myself), were also happy to see their cousin Edith, Aunt Aranka, and Uncle Hugo.

After a good night's rest, Edith talked about her possible internship. Sarah suggested the famous Toth Clinic, a gynaecology-obstetrics university institute in Budapest, where she had some connections. Edith and Sarah made arrangements by phone. Edith and Sarah, an exceptionally beautiful woman, eloquent, with a commanding appearance, always elegantly dressed, were shown around the facility by a young intern, who managed to get Edith's telephone number. Then they were ushered into the office of the director, where Edith was assured of the next summer's internship.

Everyone was impressed by Edith's vitality. Marta watched the way Edith was dressed, how she used makeup, and imitated her as well as she could. Erwin, who by then had decided that he would become a physician, was very proud of Edith, and pestered her with medical questions.

Unfortunately, the Opera and the National Philharmonic Orchestra in Budapest were closed for the summer, but there were still so many things one could do. Some theatres were open. Zsiga took the entire family for dinner to the famous open-air restaurant, Gundel, at the City Park, and Sarah succeeded in getting some tickets for the open-air theatre at Margaret Island, where Shakespeare's *A Midsummer Night's Dream* was playing. Edith went for a five o'clock tea at Margaret Island to dance with the intern from the Toth Clinic. Zsiga took the Bock family for a full day's boat ride on the *Saint Stephan* tourist cruiser on the Danube. They were taken to a typical Hungarian dinner with Gipsy music called the "Three Huszars." Sarah went to the museum with Edith and Aranka, then shopping in fashionable Vaczi Street, where they tasted delicious cakes at the nearby famous pastry shop, Gerbot.

Aranka and Hugo returned home, but Edith stayed for another week. Sad to see her go, Zsiga took Edith to the railway station.

Paul Whitman's band was playing softly on the radio as Edith sat in her little espresso bar at Wenceslas Square, sipping her coffee, wondering where the ephemeral, joyous summer vacation had gone to. It was September 16, 1935. The place was nearly empty. She had just come from the Questura, where she had registered for next year's studies. In addition to her obligatory subjects, she slipped in some clinical courses, like gynaecology-obstetrics, for she did not want to arrive at the Toth Clinic next summer as a dilettante.

On the next table lay an orphaned morning paper with a bold headline screaming: "Nuremberg Law Hits German Jews." Her hand reached out to scoop up the journal and she began reading it. She was in shock. At the yearly Nazi Party rally at Nuremberg, the new law was announced that defined "who is a Jew." Not that it involved her personally, for she did not live in Germany and knew that she was a full-blooded Jewess. Yet, the relapse into medieval conditions in a neighbouring, supposedly cultured country was incredible.

According to the new law, a single Jewish grandparent made one a Jew. The Nazis were hell-bent to give a legal definition to the question: who belongs to the Jewish "race"? Intermarriage between Jews and non-Jews was forbidden; already existing marriages were annulled unilaterally, on request. Sexual relations between Jew and non-Jew were strictly forbidden ("*Rassenschande*" or "race defilement"), and all measures to "protect the purity of the Aryan people" had to prevail. Jews were forbidden to hire female employees, lest the purity of the *Herrenvolk* (Aryan races) be contaminated with that of the *Untermenschen* (humanoids), as the Jews were portrayed. All German Jews lost their citizenships.

Edith was, of course, aware that this mania was not exclusively German. "Social Darwinism" or "scientific racism" had existed ever since a cousin of Charles Darwin's, Francis Galton, invented the term Eugenics, implying "superiority" and "inferiority" of various races. Galton's idea, Eugenics, spread fast. To demonstrate the point, since 1874, some undertakers had been transporting primitive African clans right from the jungles and exhibiting them in the zoos of Paris, London, and Berlin. These "ethnic exhibitions" had been a great success all over Europe. Sometimes these African natives were put in the same cages with the chimpanzees, to demonstrate their "inferiority." Rockefeller donated $400,000 to Ernst Rudin, the German geneticist, for his "racial research." Laws were passed and compulsory sterilization was performed on subjects in Germany, Sweden, United States (California), and Canada, mostly on uneducated Native people who were declared "mentally deficient."

The Nuremberg Laws were not surprising. Since 1933, the Nazis had been making an effort to get rid of the Jews. In 1933, they even made a pact (the Haavara Agreement) with the Zionists to transfer the German Jews to Palestine.

Edith worried how the news would affect her family, particularly her father. She placed an interurban call to Zilina but to her relief she found Hugo in his usual joking mood. With his sense of humour he assured Edith that he "has no immediate plan to divorce Aranka, the Jewess" and he was "not tempted to get involved in the near future in any interracial affairs." They had a good laugh, and Edith felt relieved.

Helene arrived the next day. Life went on as usual. The only change was a freshly painted, sparklingly clean Domoj; and Irene, the waitress, who had gained one or two kilos, had a new dress.

CHAPTER SEVEN

It was mid-afternoon on an unusually warm, sunny, October day. Back at home from her never-ending lectures, Edith had just had a refreshing shower. In her room, she shed her housecoat and lay down on top of her bed, enjoying the waxing and waning fresh air blowing in erratic gusts through the billowing curtain of the open window. Her thoughts drifted back to the introductory words of Professor Grosser, this time about embryology: "Still an underdeveloped medical field, but with a great future." He briefly reviewed the gross anatomy of the female sexual organs, then began to describe the sequential stages of gravidity. He described the menstrual cycle, ovulation, each single ripe egg — the oocyte, in medical lingo — carrying the potential of a new human life; when fertilized by the sperm, it changes its name to zygote. The process is accompanied by a complex and precise harmony of hormonal alterations and modulations, beginning with the anterior base of the brain and involving the ovaries and more, as the fertilized egg begins to germinate. This hormonal glissando lasts for forty or so weeks, ending in birth. The refined process must follow an exact, predetermined course — not unlike the libretto of a symphony. One single off-key score, and the music can end in tragedy.

As she lay on her bed, her palm grazed her nipple, still hard from the cold shower. Carnal sensations ran through her body and memories of Jan flooded her mind. The pleasurable thoughts suddenly ended when, uninvited, Vera's image forced itself into her consciousness.

Edith had so much work to do. Registered medical students had the right to attend any and every lecture — although such practice was discouraged — but without the privilege of writing any premature examinations. Yet, Edith obtained the permission of Professor Kraus, head of Gynaecology and Obstetrics, to participate in his lectures and some of the clinical proceedings.

"The special is sauerkraut with boiled potatoes and smoked sausages," announced a tired Irene with a moist brow.

"Fine, bring it to me," replied Helene.

"For me, too," said Edith. Then she turned to her friend. "What is new?"

"New? You would not be interested. Well, the prominent surgeon, Dr. Stephan Cereny, has been having a long-standing love affair with his operating room nurse; everybody knew about it."

"So?"

"His wife finally found out and left him."

"It happens every day."

"Yes, but that same nurse has had several liaisons like that."

"How come nobody tells me anything like that, but you know all the gossip in town?"

"You are not the type for it."

"And you? You are?"

"Apparently."

"But we discuss girlie things together."

"Like, for example, that you, Edith, dye your hair?"

"That is different. I always wanted to be blonde."

The food, a Czech specialty, was quite tasty.

"It would be even better with a glass of ice-cold beer."

"Can we go to the movies tomorrow evening?"

"Unfortunately not. I shall go to Klara's group tomorrow. Besides, with the added subject of gynaecology, I am very busy."

"Did you need that additional burden?"

"I did not need it but I wanted it."

"Where do you go to have your nails done?"

"Frankly, I do them myself. You know it is quite expensive; besides, all that scrubbing and formaldehyde — "

"Me, I get them done sometimes."

"And your periods?"

"No worry about that; I am celibate, you know. And yours?"

"Still Martin, but we are careful. I hear that there are some devices — "

"Yes, there are, but they are illegal to use. Professor Kraus just gave a lecture on the subject. You know how many illegal abortions there are? Even infanticides, out of desperation, are quite frequent! An American nurse, Margaret Sanger, is fighting for the rights of women to decide about their own bodies. She was arrested for giving information on contraceptive methods and devices. She worked as a nurse at a clinic in a shack town and was appalled by how many young girls were brought to the emergency rooms bleeding, dying, or dead as a result of botched-up abortions. Professor Kraus is fighting with the authorities to make contraception legal in a proper medical environment."

Edith arrived late at Klara's literary circle. A heated dissent was already in an advanced stage. In the cacophony of clashing exchange, it was difficult to follow who was saying what. The debate revolved around recent philosophical issues.

"You take Martin Heidegger — "

"No, you take him. He is a Nazi; he is one of the Old Fighter category of the Nazi Party."

"Old Fighter? What is that?"

"Yes, the ones who joined the party before or during 1933."

"Maybe so — "

"But that was the very same year when he became rector of the University of Freiburg, replacing Edmund Husserl, who retired and promoted him as his successor — "

"And he promptly broke off relations with Husserl and never again talked to him — "

"He was already famous ten years earlier, when his book *Being and Time* was published."

"It was in 1927."

"And he obtained a professorship at the University of Marburg."

"Sure. And he promptly had extramarital relations with

two of his Jewish students, Hannah Arendt and Elisabeth Blochmann."

"Jewish students? Was he not a Nazi?"

"So, he lied to both — to the Jewish students and to the Nazi Party."

"And also to his wife."

"He broke off the intimacy with the Jewish students — 'race defilement, *Rassenschande*,' you know."

"Heidegger claimed to be a Rationalist — "

"A Rationalist is supposed to respect science."

"Don't you recall his famous quotation that 'a sparrow knows more about light than a blind physicist'?"

"So, in a philosophical sense he was also an Empiricist and an Idealist to boot."

"Don't you see it? From wherever the wind blew."

"Ladies and gentlemen, friends," interrupted Klara in a loud voice. "Even though philosophy is my field of study, and I do agree with many things that were said, philosophically speaking, Heidegger is many things, but he is not an Idealist. He does not view human existence to be a spiritual issue devoid of the material, like Berkeley or Leibniz. Let us calm down. This gathering is supposed to revolve around literary matters." Hoping to change the subject, she then raised the question: "Who has seen the renewal of Anton Chekhov's *Three Sisters*?"

"I have seen it. It was gloomy," remarked one of the members.

"No, not gloomy, just Russian," interjected Edith. "I did not see the current performance but I saw it last summer in Budapest when I visited my uncle, and I also read the play. You must understand the Russian-flavoured melancholy of the impoverished Russian lower-level aristocracy. It runs throughout Russian literature."

"In the play," said somebody, "the three sisters, Olga, Masha, and Irina, are dreaming of Moscow; but the Moscow they dream about does not really exist. It is just a symbol. Their burned-out brother, Anton, is already beyond dreaming."

"Indeed," agreed Edith. "I have also been impressed by the similarities between our Kafka and Chekhov."

"Similarities?"

"Well, both of them were professionals, Kafka a lawyer, Chekhov a physician; both left their professions to be writers; both became literary giants. Both wrote about a declining culture. Neither of them could establish normal marriages or sexual lives. Both died of TB at a young age."

"Did you like the play?"

"'Like' is not the word I would use, but it is classic, unforgettable."

"And both of them were masters of the short story," somebody remarked.

There were many other unconnected issues that came under scrutiny. Like the recent death of the Czech playwright, Jaroslav Hilbert. Then Thomas Mann's *Death in Venice*, which, according to several members of the group, was dealing with Mann's own suppressed homosexuality; of the Austrian Jew, Arnold Schoenberg, with a mother from Prague, a composer and music innovator, who wrote the *Kol Nidre*, just now settled in the United States; of the Czech poet Jaroslav Seifert, born in poverty . . . his communism, his visit to the Soviet Union, and his declaration against Stalinism, for which he recruited six additional communist writers in Prague. Finally, the meeting came to an end.

It was so different! For the first time, Edith was in the world of clinical reality. She still continued, of course, her obligatory basic science studies, but the gynaecology-obstetric course confronted her for the first time with actual patients. She scrubbed up to assist surgeries and took case histories under the close supervision of the resident physician.

One of her first patients was a middle-aged woman dying of ovarian cancer. Edith was instructed to set up an intravenous tube for her. It was a mechanical task, but Edith remained sitting by the emaciated woman's side and talked to her at length. She was a Silesian woman, her husband working on construction, and she had three children. They came to see her at the official visiting hours for two hours each day, but mostly she was alone. Technicians came to her to draw blood, here and there she talked to the nurses for a few minutes, and once a day to the physician in charge. When her pain became overwhelming, she rang for the nurse. Otherwise, she was left on her own, a "public" patient sharing a room with twenty-five other patients.

As busy as Edith was, she came back to see this woman and sat at the bedside talking to her. Yes, it was different. Edith knew that the woman did not have much time left to live, and what was still ahead of her was a painful, waning spell. Edith could not stand that she was being treated simply as an object. She found herself coming back to her in the evening, bringing her some fruit, and sat beside her, sometimes with no words, just to break up her loneliness. Sometimes she brought her notes and textbooks and kept herself busy with her studies in vigil at the patient's bedside, even though she had been warned that it was not a good idea to become too personal with patients. Nevertheless, she kept up her visits till the patient's transfer to another institution. It also caused her to do some deep thinking about human existence.

CHAPTER EIGHT

The New Year's celebration had lapsed into memory by now. Helene, with Markus, Edith, and Antonin Neruda, an intern from the gynaecology clinic, spent the night dining and dancing at a small, crowded, smoke-filled club. Antonin turned out to be an excellent dancer, and had a sparkling sense of humour. The New Year, 1936, with its vague promises, unspoken expectations, and misty secrets, started off as a pending puzzle.

A warning for things to come: On the very first working day of the year, Hitler sent off a short, arrogant, purposely undiplomatic rebuff to the League of Nations answering their concern about the fate of German Jews. Hitler answered: "None of your business."

Edith left home for the university. She did not feel her usual self. She got up in the morning unsettled, with heavy head and sore muscles all over her body. *Maybe the vigorous dancing*, she thought. She could not concentrate on the lecture. Her throat was scratchy and parched. "Maybe I am getting a cold. All I need is a good hot bath and some sleep," she muttered to herself. She left the lecture and went back home. She sneezed a couple of times, she had a headache, her teeth were chattering, and she found it difficult to climb the stairs.

In her room, she undressed, throwing her clothes on the floor, and turned on the shower good and hot. She was shaking all over, had a piercing pain in her right lower chest, coughed incessantly, and felt so weak and dizzy that she wondered whether she could reach her room. The headache got violent. Edith slumped down on the floor, her head resting on her arms, which were grasping the edge of the bed.

It seemed that she fell asleep, and strange, uninvited images floated in front of her eyes. She was in Tatra on a sled, sliding down the snowy hill with uncontrollable speed toward a mountain. *Will I crash?* flashed through her mind. She was shaking but could not move; then suddenly, the mountain, like a giant throat, opened up, revealing a huge red mouth lined with sharp teeth, ready to swallow her. She felt helpless. She shrieked, her body shaking all over. She did not hear Helene and Jolana opening the door.

"I saw her leaving the lecture. She looked awful."

Then they spotted Edith's slumped body.

"My God!" cried Jolana.

They lifted her body onto her bed. "She is burning up! Do you have a thermometer?"

"I do, but I will also call my family doctor."

"Are you a nurse?" Edith did not recognize Helene, who held Edith's right arm firmly with the thermometer locked in her right armpit.

"High heavens! It is 41.5 degrees! I knew it! Her body is shaking — that means her temperature is still rising!"

Edith begun to cough, a dry, hacking cough. She was breathing rapidly; her pulse rate was fast. At one point, her body went rigid. Then she seemed to dream again. She was in a dangerous, hostile forest. Her mouth was dry, parched, but there was a rivulet. Looking upon the surface of the water, she realized that she had somehow become a deer, and there were many other deer around her. She started to run, and there were gunshots sounding again and again and again. Her heart was pounding. Suddenly, she woke up, but the gunshots continued. She realized that somebody in the neighbourhood must be hammering on some metal. Each blow reverberated with terrific pain in her head. She coughed again, bringing up rust-coloured mucus.

"Pneumonia," said the doctor to Helene, talking to her as though she were a colleague. The doctor tapped Edith's chest. "Say thirty-three," while he listened to her chest with the stethoscope. "On percussion you can hear the dullness in the right lower lobe, and increased resonance when she talks. But we must lower her temperature."

"What are we going to do?" asked Helene.

"Maybe it would be a good idea to admit her to the hospital."

"But the two of us can take care of her at home."

"Well, if you indeed can, we will wait for one day — that is, if you follow instructions." The doctor wrote three prescriptions: one for sulfonamides; another for a mixture of acetaminophen with salicylic acid, camphor, and eucalyptus, to be prepared by the pharmacist; the third for ipecacuanha-guaiacol syrup, to ease her cough. "If there is any complication, call me immediately. You can bring down her temperature with cold compresses."

Helene was shocked that on the prescription, following the doctor's signature, the doctor scribbled in Latin: "*periculum in more*," meaning, "life in danger" to ensure a speedy delivery of the drugs. This, more than anything else, made Helene realize the severity of her friend's condition.

Normal life was put on hold for Helene and Jolana, other than to care for Edith. It took them a week to break the crisis, and another week to bring her back to some degree of health; it was yet another week before Edith was almost back to her usual self. Edith could not believe how vivid her deliria had been and was amazed by the seeming "reality" of them. Of course, she fell behind with her studies but would try to make up for the lost time as best she could.

There were cheers and applause from all the tables when Edith and Helene entered the Domoj after three weeks' absence. "The applause is all for you, Helene," said Edith, her eyes sparkling with tears.

In late January, King George V of the United Kingdom, a firm opponent of Hitler, passed away. George V, one of the fifty-four grandchildren of Queen Victoria, was the one who renounced the Sachs-Coburg-Gotha German family name of the British rulers, changing it to "Windsor" in 1917. At his spectacular funeral, a German cousin, Charles Edward, Duke of Albany and Head of the Sachs-Coburg-Gotha family, demonstratively wore his high-ranking Nazi SA uniform (SA: *Sicherheit Abteilung* — Security Department), decorated with a swastika. The throne then went to son Edward VIII; there had been a lifelong hostility between father and son.

Edward VIII had been raised by a male "nanny," Hans Heinlein, for more than ten years, who taught him fluent German. Henlein's influence may well have been the root of Edward's bizarre sexuality. After his coronation, Edward insisted on marrying the twice-divorced Wallis Simpson, which purportedly led to his stepping down from the throne in less than one year. The truth is that security forces in the United Kingdom, and even in the United States, J. Edgar Hoover in particular, were concerned about Edward VIII's loyalty. Mrs. Simpson's love affair with the then German Ambassador, Herr Joachim Ribbentrop, was still going on. Edward's good friend was Oswald Mosley, head of the British Nazi Party, a personal friend of Hitler's. Shortly after his abdication, Edward himself visited Hitler.

In early 1936, Hitler had a dilemma. The Olympics were coming to Germany, a most valuable propaganda tool, costing billions. Along with that came thousands of visiting journalists and countless numbers of tourists. The image of Nazi Germany became an all-important matter. Hitler forbade all visible signs of anti-Semitism, along with a "temporary" abolishment of all anti-Semitic posters and all billboards demanding the boycott of Jewish businesses.

Hitler, dressed in his Nazi uniform, wearing his precious iron cross — which he had received from his Jewish superior in World War I, Lt. Hugo Gutmann, who later had to settle in the United States — opened the Winter Olympics in early February, hoping for German victories in all categories, to prove Aryan racial superiority.

Hitler could not stand to be seen as weak. March came, and with Nazi fanfare, he broke the Versailles Peace Treaty when, with spectacular military showmanship, he remilitarized the Rhineland.

At the same time, the search was on to find one single Jewish athlete to represent Germany in the Games, just to oppose possible troublemakers who would say that German Jews were excluded from participating. They were lucky. A German Jewess, Helene Meyer, actually from a Jewish father but a Christian mother, who lived in Offenbach, Germany, was an outstanding fencing champion. Brought up in the Jewish faith, she, according to the Nuremberg Law, was a full Jewess and had lost her German citizenship. She went to live with her uncle in San Francisco. Blonde, tall, she had been a German patriot all along. She was contacted by the German consulate, and she was more than ready to return to Germany, if she could get back her German citizenship.

The Olympic Village was built by Albert Speer, Hitler's favourite architect. Goebbels invented the spectacular Olympic marathon run with the Olympic flame, brought from Athens to Berlin. This practice was put in action for the first time. Richard Strauss, in his enthusiasm, composed the "Olympic Hymn." The German population was warned to refrain from eating eggs, to ensure that the tourists would have enough. Also, they were forbidden to discuss anti-Semitism for the duration of the Olympics. A Love Garden was built near the Olympic village, where German girls were encouraged to mingle — and more — with athletes; in the event of pregnancy, the State would look after mother and child. Twenty thousand pigeons were released, and huge Nazi flags were hung everywhere. The only country that boycotted the Olympics was Ireland.

Just before the Olympics, on July 17, the Spanish Civil War broke out.

Edith was in Budapest, working at the Toth Clinic as an intern. Many times, she remained at the clinic overnight to participate in deliveries, or because she was chosen to be "second assistant" for early-morning surgeries. She enjoyed her internship very much, and she was recognized for her extensive knowledge of gynaecology and obstetrics. What they were expecting was a total beginner. Still, there was time for all kinds of cultural events, dancing, and social life. Uncle Zsiga and his entire family, particularly Erwin, were so proud of Edith. And, of course, she was listening to the radio reports of the Olympics.

In women's fencing, the gold medal was won by a Jewish Hungarian, Ilona Schacherer–Elek, Helene Meyer got the silver, and the Jewish Austrian Ellen Preis got the bronze medal. All three medals in women's fencing were won by Jewesses. At the medal ceremony, only Helene Meyer gave the Nazi salute with raised arm. She returned to the United States after the Games and remained a German Nazi patriot, even though some of her family members were murdered in the concentration camps.

Hungary did well, all in all: At the combined medal count, Hungary was in third place. Germany came first with thirty-three medals, and the United States came in second. Ending up in first place was most important for the Nazis.

In early September, Edith went back to Zilina. They celebrated the Jewish High Holidays together. Neither Edith nor her family were very religious, but a deep belonging to Judaism prevailed in the Kohn and Bock families. Only the grandparents kept a kosher kitchen. But their firm Jewishness and support of the dream of an independent Jewish State as promised in the Balfour Declaration had very deep roots. Edith recalled the little blue-white box in Grandma's kitchen to collect pennies for the Cause. That is why the family rejoiced that the British Peel Commission left for Palestine in the same month, and eventually, came up with the recommendation of a two-state solution.

After the holidays, Edith returned to Prague.

Nevertheless, the year was not over yet. Klara's biweekly meeting in October rejoiced that Eugene O'Neill had won the well-deserved Nobel Prize for literature. Everyone recalled Edith's remarks the previous year about O'Neill's eligibility.

In early November, Hitler made a pact with Mussolini, the famous "Rome-Berlin Axis," tying the two nations into a close alliance, which was followed within a few days by the Anti-Comintern Pact, drawing Japan into the treaty as well. Soon, before the year's end, Japan attacked China.

CHAPTER NINE

Edith's studies now became a race against the momentum of the gathering political storm. Who will win, who will lose? Few people doubted that a devastating war could still be avoided. Edith searched for means and ways to shorten her studies, but her chances to do so were limited by university regulations. She was now at a stage of her curriculum where clinical subjects—such as surgery, internal medicine, neurology, and the like—became the focus of her program. All she could do was to complete her internships on the required courses during her vacation time. Her private life vanished; she studied day and night. Besides the lectures, she did voluntary night and weekend duties, mainly in the emergency room, hoping these optional activities might be recognized by the university. As she toiled, the European political situation was rapidly deteriorating.

But not everyone shared a pessimistic view. Among them—surprisingly—was Hugo, who no longer could live in his dark world of landscape, and switched somehow into an existence of denial. He found that he had accumulated a sizable amount of cash and persuaded himself that the best investment would be real estate and to build a luxurious family home. It would always survive, he reasoned, and eventually would remain in the family. After all, Jewish life in the Diaspora had all along been marked by ups and downs. Yes, life itself may be in danger; cash, jewellery, movable assets may be lost; but a house is there forever. Currently, real estate prices were at their lowest level, and the construction sector struggled with unemployment; therefore, to build a house was a tempting investment. Nobody close to Hugo would disagree with him, probably because they feared to plunge him into a new episode of despair. Edith was surprised but shared Hugo's opinion, and, if anything, she encouraged him to go ahead with his plan. What was the alternative? What was the difference?

Klara's literary circle, meeting once every two weeks, remained Edith's only relaxation. Edith was looking forward to tonight's gathering. In opposition to Klara, the majority of the members insisted on altering the original line of discussion. Instead of investigating the enchanting literary issues, there was a crying need to grasp the current events that involved everyone's lives.

"But the facts are all over the radio and have become a media frenzy," Klara tried to argue.

"They are giving us the facts, yes, but the illumination of the causes and their dynamics is more important than the sheer facts."

"And what would they be, in your opinion?"

"The reasons go back well before the Great War," opined somebody.

"You think so? Explain it to us, then."

"Well, then, I must go back before the 1850s and start with a seemingly remote subject.

"John D. Rockefeller's father was a travelling quack. He used 'rock oil,' as it was called then, for liniment. I am talking about rock oil in the Western world, for oil was known in the East long before that. But the main business in Pennsylvania at that time was raising cattle. Cattle need salt, and although they had some saltwater springs, they had been contaminated by rock oil. What a nuisance!

"In 1854, Samuel Kier began to produce and export barrels of oil; the oil was used as a light lubricant and, by snake-oil quacks, for liver disease and for liniment. There was not much demand for it. A journalist, George Bissel, sent some oil to Professor Benjamin Silliman at Yale for analysis.

"When Edward Drake drilled for oil, the price fell precipitously. John Rockefeller did well, however, because he owned the railways for export. This is when William Wright's book on refining oil appeared, and the next year, the Humboldt

Refinery opened. In 1868, Rockefeller established the Standard Oil Company. In 1876, Nikolaus August Otto invented a two-stroke internal combustion motor. Ten years later, Karl Benz, another German engineer, modified it to a four-stroke engine, requiring oil products.

"Meanwhile, in 1888, D'Arcy found oil in Mesopotamia [later called Iraq]. In 1893, Rudolf Diesel developed the very economical Diesel engine. By 1903, Ford was pouring out Model T automobiles, and in the very same year, Orville and Wilbur Wright sent their first planes into the air. In 1911, Winston Churchill, then First Lord of Admiralty, was warned by his experts that unless the British fleet could reach a speed of twenty-five knots per hour, the British hegemony on the sea would be lost. In the same year, the Germans, demonstratively, sent a warship to Morocco. Still in the same year, 1911, Marshall Foch of France declared to journalists that the newly invented airplane was just a toy and would never gain any military significance.

"By then, the German submarines were running on Diesel engines. A panic arose about a worldwide oil shortage. The Germans, who had no oil of their own, began to build the Baghdad–Berlin railway, and the Americans began to produce new tanks, requiring a lot of fuel. During the Great War, the British had sent an MI6 agent to the Middle East, an ingenious woman, Gertrude Bell, who was assisted by two agents, one of whom was Lawrence of Arabia, who tried, unsuccessfully, to raise an Arab revolt against the Ottoman Empire. Gertrude Bell was busy in Iraq. The other agent, John Philby, worked for himself, making friends with the Wahhabi tribe and with King Ibn Saud. In 1933, having been dismissed, John Philby turned Muslim and persuaded his friend King Ibn Saud to search for oil in the desert. The King approved the plan, and Abdullah Philby contacted Charles Crane in Chicago, who sent his engineer, Karl Twitchell. Twitchell in 1936 found huge oil deposits in Saudi Arabia. Standard Oil bought them immediately. And this, ladies and gentlemen, took place in less than one hundred years."

"Also," remarked somebody, "oil is used for generating

electricity."

"And add to it that Germany lost in 1919 whatever few colonies in Africa they had, and they have no crude oil of their own."

"But they developed the Fischer–Tropsch method of producing oil from coal."

"Not very economical. One ton of coal yields only two hundred litres of fuel."

"And this will decide British politics."

"That will be tough on the Jews in Palestine."

"You are telling me that Hitler wants to turn Europe into a German Colony?"

"Well, Poland has oil; so do the Soviet Union and Rumania."

"So, we are the victims of technology and a madman."

"Now I understand why the British are so keen to please the Arabs."

"It is all about economy."

"What does the poverty-stricken Palestinian Jew have to offer the British?"

"Nothing will surprise me. War is unavoidable."

Soon after Klara's unintended "political meeting," Edith and Helene dined at the Domoj, sharing a table with Teresa Janovic and Gisella Herzikova, by then advanced political science students. Both were deeply involved in a fiery conversation about the current political situation, as were so many people in Prague. Teresa, always somewhat of a Pollyanna, emphasized the military might of Czechoslovakia and the unshakable East and West alliances.

Gisella was doubtful. "You must remember, Teresa, that the current British leadership, Prime Minister Neville Chamberlain and Foreign Secretary Lord Halifax, are terrified of war. Two years ago, on the invitation of Nazi Propaganda Minister Joseph Goebbels, Lord Halifax, then Baldwin's Minister of War, was invited 'privately' to Nazi Germany. Halifax met Hitler and came back praising the Nazi system. 'Fantastic,' he reported, 'and Hitler also keeps the Soviets in check and has put the communists and their leaders in concentration camps.'

"Neville Chamberlain, a self-confessed anti-Semite — which he made abundantly clear in a letter to his sister — is against war, no matter what. He appointed Lord Halifax to become his Foreign Secretary. That does not look well for us, does it? Only Churchill is opposing him but he has no power."

"Did Lord Halifax say anything about the desperate situation of the German Jews?" asked Edith.

"Not a word."

It had been a bad year for Jews everywhere — as if there were ever any good ones — and still worse to come. There were pogroms in Poland. Rumania wanted all Jews to leave the country. All of the Soviet leaders who initiated the Jewish Province, Birobidjan, were arrested, and the province "disappeared," leaving the Jewish population of Birobidjan just a tiny minority. This was the year of Stalin's "Great Purge," when 750,000 people were murdered. The highly anti-Semitic Slovakian Party and its "Hlinka Guard" got stronger each year.

Franco's forces in Spain executed 35,000 people. Among the captured was Arthur Koestler, facing execution, but he escaped at the last moment. He later described his harrowing experience in his book *Dialogue with Death*.

Hitler gave a great speech in Nuremberg about the need for German "*Lebensraum*" (living space), implying colonization of Eastern Europe.

A German "Judische Auswanderung Bureau" (Jewish Emigration Office) was opened under the directorship of Adolf Eichmann. He even travelled to Palestine and negotiated with Zionist and Arab leaders but he was expelled by the British.

Masaryk, who had given over the presidency of Czechoslovakia to Edvard Beneš two years previously, passed away.

A scared Edith went home and cried into her pillow all night. What will the future bring? Can she finish her studies before disaster hits?

CHAPTER TEN

Edith was delighted. Most of her internships were recognized by the university, shortening her studies by eight weeks. Her volunteer work at the emergency room, all those exhausting weekends, was not officially acknowledged. However, she learned more medicine there than anywhere else, what with the variety of cases overflowing the ER, some of which she witnessed and others she treated. There is nothing more educational in the medical field than what the ER offers, with its hectic involvement in whatever life throws its way.

Klara's meeting was coming up once again. Edith wavered as to whether she should attend. The last gathering had upset her, even though it was educational. Finally, she decided to go. *I might not stay*, she compromised.

Klara, to prevent a repetition of the last get-together, announced to the usual audience that she had a surprise waiting.

"I am your elected president. Therefore, it is my privilege to alter our cultural program. If you did not like it, on the closure of the evening you may have my resignation.

"Tonight we will have a 'lady's concert.' All of the composers you will hear, all of the musicians who will play, are women — and all of them are Czechs."

A small murmur arose while the valet began to distribute some small mimeographed sheets. They also noted that Klara's piano had been moved into the meeting room.

> *PROGRAM - HOUSE CONCERT:*
> *KATERINA EMINGEROVA: Polonaise for Violin and Piano.*

AUGUSTA AUSPITZ-KOLAROVA: Scherzo Fantastique Op.2.

-Intermission-

AGNES TYRRELL: String Quartet in G Major for Chamber Orchestra.
Music by Student Volunteers of Prague Conservatorium:
Piano: ELIZA JAHONOV
Violin: ANNA SVOBODA
Cello: LUDMILLA KURTZ
Clarinet: HANNA DUSCHAK

"You have the program in your hand. The volunteer students of the Prague Conservatorium have agreed to the musical evening, and have been practising every evening after a short notice of ten days."

A spontaneous, vigorous applause sounded as the four young women walked into the room, three of them carrying musical instruments.

"Just a few words about the composers. Katerina Emingerova and Augusta Auspitz were students of Bedrich Smetana; both of them were born in Prague. Katerina began to compose at age thirteen, and Augusta began to learn piano at age five in Smetana's school. Agnes Tyrrell was born and lived in Brno, Moravia; she gave her first recital at age nine. All these lady composers lived in the nineteenth century. Emingerova also pioneered women's rights, advanced women composers, and wrote articles in magazines such as *Female World*, *New Women*, and the like."

While Klara was speaking, in the background, as usual, the musicians were tuning their instruments. Then all turned silent, and suddenly the enchanting music filled the room with magic.

For all, this house concert remained a rare and blissful memory in a violent world seething with hate, wanton rancour, and ominous potential.

They did not have to wait long. Hitler commanded Konrad Henlein, the head of the renamed German Sudeten Party, to Berlin and ordered him to demand complete Sudeten autonomy. That created an upheaval in Czechoslovakia. In February 1938, Hitler instructed Chancellor Kurt Schuschnigg of Austria to come for a meeting at his Bavarian home, Berchtesgaden, and demanded that a plebiscite be held to join Austria with Greater Germany. Schuschnigg, still hoping that the Austrians would choose to remain autonomous, agreed. But the polling never took place, as the German army entered Austria on March 11, 1938, to the delight of the Austrian population. There were celebrations all over Austria.

Schuschnigg was arrested and put in a concentration camp. The power went into the hands of Arthur Seyss-Inquart, the head of the Austrian Nazi Party. He held a ballot, and more than 99 percent of the population voted for joining Germany. Tens of thousands of Jews were arrested, and large crowds of jeering and taunting Austrians watched the Jews, who were forced to scrub the pavements of Vienna with toothbrushes. Many Jews were put in concentration camps, while many escaped to Hungary, where they lived illegally. The roads of freedom were blocked for the Jews. And the Western powers? They did nothing.

The Nazis had not even had time to gobble up Austria when, in April 1938, Konrad Henlein openly demanded separation and an independent German-Sudeten autonomy in Czechoslovakia. Few people knew that Hitler, more than a year before, had made secret plans with his generals for the occupation of Czechoslovakia.

Hitler gave speeches in which he maintained that the German minority was facing "annihilation" by the Czechs. He also encouraged Slovakia to demand separation and independence from the Czechs, something that appealed greatly to the Slovaks.

In July 1938, F.D. Roosevelt called a meeting concerning the doomed European Jewry. The meeting started on the wrong foot. Canada and Switzerland refused to attend the meeting. Pope Pius XII declined. Finally, France agreed to host the meeting in Evian. As a condition of the majority, the word "Jew" was not allowed to be used; instead, the code word "refugee" was employed. None of the participants would agree to increase their quota for immigrants. The British did not want to upset the oil-rich Arabs by opening Palestine for Jewish immigration. The Evian Conference was a total failure.

Hitler was well informed of the military weakness of the Western powers, of the widely shared disinclination of the British and French public to enter a new war, of the United States' isolationism, of the poverty and unemployment due to the Great Depression, of the widespread fear of communism; all of this encouraged Hitler.

There had been a silent impulse toward sympathy for Nazism by the masses, as well by British leadership, starting from King Edward VIII, to the government leaders; and the insatiable British need for possession of oil resources fed the flame. Hitler did not need any spies to acquire this knowledge. It sufficed to listen to the BBC, or to read the foreign press, with messages like Neville Chamberlain's radio broadcast to the public at large: "How terrible it is that we should be digging trenches and trying on gas masks here because of a quarrel in a faraway country between people of whom we know nothing . . ."

The previous indifference of Hitler's enemies to his breaking the Versailles Treaty, their reaction to his remilitarizing the Rhineland, and to swallowing up Austria, translated in Hitler's mind to: "Do what you want." And he did just that.

The seventy-year-old Neville Chamberlain, on his own request, went to see Hitler, hat in hand, at Berchtesgaden on September 15, 1938. The forty-nine-year-old dictator did not receive him at the airport on arrival but gave him a list of his demands. Chamberlain returned to London and, a week later, flew once again to Bad Godesberg. This time, Hitler kept him waiting for hours and let Chamberlain know that meanwhile his demands had been increased. Chamberlain agreed but asked Hitler to sign a piece of paper about a potential peace agreement.

Waving it as a flag on his return to London, he made a declaration that still rings in the ears of many: "Peace in our time! Peace with honour."

On September 29, 1938, Chamberlain flew to Germany, this time to Munich. The French prime minister, Édouard Daladier, Mussolini, Chamberlain, and Hitler had a conference. Chamberlain legally accepted Mussolini's rights to Ethiopia. Hitler increased his demands yet further. A complete ring around the remaining Czech nation now became Independent Sudetenland, that is, Greater Germany. These territories contained all of the Czech defences and her heavy industries. A piece of Czech territory went to Poland, another piece to Hungary. In return, Hitler promised that he would tolerate whatever remained from the Czech nation. The Czechs were not invited to the meeting. That was the Munich Dictate. One can imagine how all these stories were heralded in minute detail in a mesmerized German media — and what it did to an already enchanted nation.

Chamberlain flew home and was received as a hero by the cheering masses, by King George VI, and by Parliament.

The British did everything in their power to make the Czechs accept the "deal." President Beneš of Czechoslovakia resigned on October 5 and went into exile in London. The presidency was taken over by Emil Hacha, approved by the Nazis.

This was the year when Hitler ordered that all the mentally ill and those with incurable illnesses, representing a "burden on the nation," should be "euthanized." The German medical profession, under the spell of the Nazis, with a newly altered code of ethics, agreed with this policy, and in the next few years, some 270,000 psychiatric patients were murdered.

To end the year, on November 7, in Paris, a desperate seventeen-year-old Jewish boy, Herschel Grynszpan, shot and killed the German diplomat, Ernst vom Rath. This sparked in Germany the "Crystal Night," an orgy of violence against Jews. Almost one thousand Jews were killed, many ended up in concentration camps, more than 190 synagogues were burned down, and thousands of Jewish businesses and properties were looted and destroyed. The Jewish community was fined millions of Reichsmarks for the damages. What a year that was!

CHAPTER ELEVEN

Edith was crying bitterly into her pillow, this time throughout the night. Beyond consolation, her shoulders were shaking, tears flowing, as she sobbed. She was in the second semester of the fifth and last year of her studies, all her examinations passed successfully, just waiting for three months to pass till her graduation from medical school. It was late March of 1939 when Hitler broke the Munich Agreement, signed by himself six months previously, and marched into the remaining tiny Czech territory. The hamstrung Hacha remained the president, but the power was in the hands of the SS. Emboldened by the Nazi move, Jozef Tiso declared Slovakia an independent state. A double blow. This move cut Edith off from her family in Zilina, which was now in Slovakia, and shattered her lifelong dream of becoming a physician.

Still, Edith was lucky. Thousands of students and professors were arrested and taken to concentration camps, most of them never to be heard of again. Suicide among Czechs and Jews was rampant. The Germans were drunk on their "victory." A German physician, a dunce in Nazi uniform, burst into the operating room of the famous professor Jirassek during surgery, shouting "Heil Hitler," and making the Nazi salute, declaring: "I am in charge here." The barbarian occupiers created havoc and horror in Prague. Despair took over the city, and in the confusion, all felt that the unexpected catastrophe would wipe out the entire nation.

In the morning, with red eyes, Edith, a shadow of her former self, decided to go to the Questura to attempt to bargain for recognition of her time spent in the emergency room, which would make her eligible for graduation. Instead, they placed a stamp in her Report Book: "*Abgangerzeugniss*" — "Leaving

Certificate," snuffing out five years of hard work and obliterating a dearly desired dream with a single rubber stamp.

Her arteries throbbing in her neck, Edith went to see Professor Grosser. A gloomy Grosser, grasping the despair of his worthy student, uttered: "I am totally helpless, Edith. I should not even see you here. Go home to your parents. Save your life. I am truly sorry." Grosser was not a Nazi. An agonizing pain ran through Edith's body, in her temples, felt all the way down to her loins, reminiscent of the birth pains she had witnessed in the gynaecology clinic.

She ran to the emergency room, wanting to talk to somebody. There, she found a madhouse. Czech policemen and ambulance drivers were bringing in more and more patients, some alive, some dead or dying — suicide cases, some barely alive; heart attack patients. The staff were all running around in circles. She found the head nurse.

"Go away, Edith, the SS are all over the place."

"And you?"

"I am not afraid of them. But you go, and go right now!"

Till then, it had not occurred to Edith that her very life was in immediate danger, and, in her bitterness, she did not care.

Maybe I will find somebody in the Domoj, thought Edith. The Domoj was nearly empty, except for two Sudeten bus drivers sitting at a table.

"Go away," whispered a distraught Irene. "Go away *now*. They just arrested two students . . ."

Edith ran into Jolana at home. "Go home to Zilina, immediately," Jolana said. "I shall help you pack."

Edith was numb. They packed most of Edith's things, some of which she did not care for, but she could not part from her Sobotta anatomy atlas and her white coat.

"What about Helene?"

"She was here looking for you. She left for Bratislava. She told me that she would call you in Zilina."

The train station was swarming with SS soldiers but they concentrated on catching young, military-age men. As so many times before, Edith took the train. Few people dared to do the same. She was left alone.

Frantic thoughts overcame Edith in the empty compartment of the train. No more lectures, no more Questura, no more Helene, Klara, or Domoj. No more white coat, no more bleaching of her hair, no more lipstick, silk stockings, Mitsouko; no more concerts and invigorating discussions; no more smiles; no dancing.

Yes, she thought; *yes, we all have to die*. Once Freud was asked, "What is the purpose of life?" He answered: "The purpose of life is death." *But there is death and death*, thought Edith.

Cicero, in his essay on old age, "De Senectute," wrote an analogy: "When one tears down an unripe apple, it is a violent act, the whole branch is ripped off; but the ripe apple falls in your palm, just by touching it. Thus the young die by violence, the old from maturity."

Yes, contemplated Edith, *it is different to die after a fulfilled life in peace, surrounded by a caring family and attentive physicians, and another thing to perish in young age, wasted, starved, and humiliated in the inhuman milieu of a concentration camp.*

She went on thinking. *What is death? Giving up our precious consciousness. What is consciousness, after all? It is a mélange of past and present. But the past, no matter how beautiful it may have been, is gone anyway. And, if the present is just pain, death is a relief. The ancient Greeks imagined that on passing, we must drink from the water of Lethe, so that we forget what is gone. The future? The future does not exist, because by the time it arrives, it is already present, and the next split second, it is past already.*

Surprisingly, Edith had no trouble getting through the border between the Czech Protectorate and the newly born Slovakia. Nobody knew that she was coming home, so nobody was waiting for her. This brought renewed tears to her eyes as she recalled her cheerful arrival only two years ago.

Aranka screamed with joy when Edith stepped into their new home—Hugo had made his investment. She embraced Edith and did not let her go. "My dear, darling daughter, *moja dusha*! I worried about you night and day! Nothing else matters than that you are at home! The diploma? The hell with it!" She could not stop kissing Edith. To her surprise, Edith, too, felt happy. And so did her father, her brothers, the entire Kohn and Bock family. Millennia of persecution have taught Jews to live with this kind of priority.

"What is happening in the family?" asked Edith.

"Really, not much. Your Cousin Zsuzsa finally left with an underground Zionist ship to Palestine. Imagine — they were on that tiny crowded boat on the Mediterranean for forty days, constantly harassed by the British Navy, time and time again barely getting away. A second cousin, Braun Pista from Bratislava, was on the ship, too. Somehow they got lucky and drifted close to the shore at Natanya, and they all swam to the shore. Their sole worldly possessions on arrival were wet swimsuits. But Hagana, the Jewish underground was waiting for them, and before the British military arrived, all of them were hidden, Zsuzsa in a kibbutz, and Braun Pista with a family in Tel Aviv."

"Wonderful! And the rest of the family?"

"Uncle Bela tried the same or a similar route. He went to Budapest at first, stayed for some time with Uncle Zsiga, then he travelled to Bucharest, where he lost all his saved-up money on horse races. He came home without a cent and without any hope of leaving the country again."

"Not surprising. Pity that his wife and daughter, Judith, too, were cheated out of the chance to immigrate to Palestine."

"And now we are awaiting the new Slovak anti-Semitic Law to come. But nothing matters — just that you are with us."

Earlier in the year, the Wagner–Rogers Bill was put to a vote; it proposed to send 20,000 German children to the United States. The bill asked for temporary shelter for these children during the war. The bill was defeated because it was felt that it would not be right to show favouritism to one ethnic group over the others.

The *Peel Commission Report* suggested a two-nation solution for Palestine; it was accepted by the Jews but rejected by the Arabs. In May 1939, the British came out with the *White Paper*, essentially closing Jewish immigration to Palestine. With that, the last hope of the European Jewry was gone. Hitler set fire to the house of the Jew, and the rest of the world blocked all the exit doors.

Laci, Zolo, and another cousin, Paul, were determined to leave home. They had unconfirmed news about joining the Czechoslovakian Legion, which Edvard Beneš was organizing from London.

"It breaks our hearts, you know, but we could not interfere with whatever they do. They decided to go. But they are just mere children!"

In early May 1939, the boys said goodbye and, with Hugo's help and finances, they crossed the border into Poland. It was not quite as simple as it sounds, but they were finally on their way.

Helene called from Bratislava. She soon was leaving for Palestine on an illegal ship. She begged Edith to come with her. But Edith could not bear separation from her parents, so much more because the boys were planning to leave the family. Edith just could not add more sorrow to her parents and leave the two of them alone, facing vicious times to come. Both Edith and Helene could not stop crying.

In midsummer 1939, the SS *St. Louis*, a German passenger liner, was heading to the United States with approximately one thousand German Jews. Each had a valid immigration visa to enter the United States, but the visas would become valid only on the first of August. Being on the sea one month too early, they would stop in the Dominican Republic and wait for their immigration visas to mature. For that reason, they also had a Dominican visiting visa. When they arrived at the shores of the Dominican Republic, these visiting visas were withdrawn. They tried everything in their power to validate their U.S. immigration visas for immediate maturity. The U.S. authorities would not hear of it.

The American Jewish Community offered to cover all expenses and asked the U.S. authorities to deport these people to Ellis Island until their immigration visas became valid. This, too, was turned down. Canada would not accept them, nor would any other country, not even temporarily.

In desperation, people began to commit suicide on the ship. The German captain was supposed to return to Hamburg but he decided to beach the ship on the shore of England. At that point England, Belgium, and France offered shelter, each accepting one-third of the passengers. Those who were accepted by England were lucky. The other two-thirds ended up eventually in German concentration camps and did not survive. Hitler was thrilled: "See, nobody wants the Jews."

Another illegal ship, the *Salvador II*, with Uruguayan registration —a barely moving tub with a capacity of thirty to forty people, no compass, and no life jackets—was heading to Palestine carrying 327 passengers; it left on December 15, 1940. It sailed into a storm and sank. Two hundred and four people, including sixty-six children, died. Of the survivors, sixty-three were sent back to the Germans, and the rest of them were jailed by the British in Atlit, Palestine.

The Slovaks copied everything that the Nazis did to the Jews. They turned out to be faithful allies of Hitler. True, they lost some territory to Hungary—a gift of Hitler's to the Hungarians—but those domains were populated by the hated Hungarians and by the despised Jews, and it was ultimately not a significant loss for the Slovaks, except for the property of the Jews. The remainder of Slovakia, with 90,000 Jews (of whom 10,000 escaped to live illegally in Hungary) was ruled by sixteen Nazi Catholic priests. Andrej Hlinka had worked diligently since the nineteen-twenties to set up the Hlinka Guards, which eventually became the equivalent of the German SS. The head of the Slovak Party and president of Slovakia was Monseigneur Jozef Tiso; his prime minister was Vojtech Tuka, a priest.

No help was coming to the Slovak Jews; the anti-Semitism of the new regime got worse and worse.

One year later, on September 1, 1941, the "Jewish Code" was instituted in Slovakia, obliging Jews to wear a yellow star on their clothing. Jews were not allowed to own any form of property, and work camps were set up for forced labour.

Uncle Sandor, with his wife, Sara, escaped to Hungary. Uncle Zsiga took care of them, supplying them with forged papers, and they lived in Buda, in Zsiga's cottage. Zsiga also made an arrangement with his influential immediate neighbour, Tivadar Homonnay, a member of the Hungarian Senate, to open a secret door at the fence for them, to escape, if needed.

CHAPTER TWELVE

While Edith herself would not hear of leaving her parents in Zilina, it became her mission to instigate and to prepare the escape of her brothers, Laci and Zolo, and Cousin Paul to relative "safety" in Poland. Through the tireless perseverance of Edith and the insistence of Hugo, the three boys got over the border just a few months before the Nazis attacked Poland – with whom Hitler had a signed a ten-year Friendship Agreement; an act that sparked World War II.

The three boys, like many of their fellow Czech refugees, were eager to join the forces fighting the Nazis.

Well before the end of the Great War and the proclamation of Czechoslovakia in 1918, Tomas Masaryk and Edvard Beneš had set up a tough Czech fighting unit that battled valiantly alongside the Allied Forces. The Czech combatants were trained by the French Foreign Legion, which passed over to them their well-recognized endurance, esprit de corps, and unbending self-sacrifice.

When President Beneš resigned and went into exile in London in 1938, after the Nazi occupation, he did not waste any time before setting up the original Czechoslovak Legion, renewing the camaraderie with the Foreign Legion. Once again, the Foreign Legion took charge of training the Czechs.

The mystique of the dauntless French Foreign Legion is commonly known to the public at large from books, films, and legend. Less recognized is the close tie between the Foreign Legion and the Czechoslovak Legion.

This became known to Laci, Zolo, Cousin Paul, and many other Czech refugees in Warsaw, when they signed up with the Foreign Legion at the French Embassy. They were sent to a camp nearby, and each time the number of volunteers reached 150, they were sent to Lyons.

In Lyons, Laci experienced for the first time the tough life of the legionnaires. While there, Laci developed a vicious toothache. He reported this to the corporal, who sent four legionnaires with fixed bayonets to escort Laci to the nearest dentist. They held him motionless in the dentist chair, and, without any anaesthesia, after several unsuccessful attempts, the dentist removed the tooth. Laci was escorted back to the barracks, had some swill for supper, and was housed in a cattle wagon. They were on their way to Marseille. This was how Laci learned about the less glorious side of the Foreign Legion.

In Marseille, an ancient Mediterranean port city established by the Greeks and Phoenicians, the unit was placed in a bedbug-infested fortress where they slept on straw-filled mattresses. Next morning, they had to shed all civilian clothes, and were issued well-worn fatigues. The civilian clothes were bought up by a bunch of dealers for a pittance. After peeling potatoes and sweeping the yard, mingling by then with a large number of Legionnaires from a wide variety of countries, many of them escapees from prisons and assorted misfits, they boarded the cattle deck of a ship, moving slowly to Oran, Algeria, and, without rest, by train to Sidi–Bel–Abbes, the headquarters of the Foreign Legion.

Here, they were given new uniforms, rifles, ammunition belts, heavy boots, field flasks, and a twelve-foot-long, ten-inch-wide cloth that they were supposed to wear around their waists. Each of them received a number (Laci's number was 84359), and their names no longer existed. Without any questions asked, they got vaccinated, which made everyone sick, then left for the garrison at Saida. It was a training camp near the Atlas Mountains and the desert. Reveille at 5:00 a.m., breakfast, then training. They were taught how to fold their uniforms. They went on forty-kilometre marches wearing overcoats on the red-hot desert sands, with ninety-pound backpacks; a cast-iron weight in the ammunition belt; a rifle with bayonet; and two pints of water in their field flasks, which they were not allowed to drink (it was checked on return). When a comrade collapsed, his neighbour had to carry his rifle and ammunition belt. The overcoats became wringing wet from sweat, allegedly "keeping them cool and preventing dehydration" — in summer on the Sahara.

In his autobiography, Laci described two incidents. Two friends got into an argument. One picked up a chair and hit the other on the head, who died on the spot. At his funeral, the officer said: "He was a good soldier; his uniforms were always nicely folded." End of the story. On another occasion, a German corporal kept teasing "Andrew," a Czech giant of a man. When Andrew had had enough, he picked up the German corporal and threw him out the first-floor window. The man died, and, again, no more words were spoken of the event.

It was a fortunate thing that Laci and Zolo were still able to correspond with their parents in Zilina. They learned that Hugo had lost his business, the new house was confiscated, and, a little while later, the "Jewish Code" came into existence in Slovakia. From then on, they had to wear yellow stars on their clothes and do hard manual labour. Edith worked as a physician with a group of girls doing such forced labour; she maintained their morale and she was loved by her confreres.

In August 1939, Hitler and Stalin made a "non-aggression pact." Like two poker players both knowing that the other is cheating, Molotov and Ribbentrop sat at the table with pretended honesty. The only bilaterally accepted part of the agreement was how the two divided Poland among each other. Stalin gained time; Hitler avoided fighting simultaneously on both the Eastern and Western fronts.

On September first, Hitler attacked Poland, and World War II was on. Chamberlain still hoped that the war could come to a halt; there were secret negotiations; Chamberlain was tempted to give up Suez — even Gibraltar — to the Italians, and return the prewar African colonies to Germany.

Hitler visited Prague, the capital of the "Czech Protectorate," stayed in Prague Castle, and, ironically, ordered Vaclav Talich, the conductor of the Czech Philharmonic Orchestra, to come to Berlin to perform for a Nazi audience Smetana's *My Country*, a group of symphonic poems of the Czechs.

The German troops were bombing Warsaw and were killing thousands of fleeing civilians on the highways with their dive bombers. When the occupation was complete, they murdered innumerable Polish people, targeting mainly the intelligentsia and army officers. The bloody task was committed by a newly set up "*Einsatzgruppe*" (murder squad) under the authority of Heinrich Himmler, Reichsfuehrer and head of the SS. It was performed under the command of Reinhard Heydrich, with the devoted participation of Dieter Wisliceny and Otto Ohlenberg. Adolf Eichmann assisted in setting up mass transport to forced labour camps.

The Soviets, according to the Pact with Germany, also took their share of Eastern Poland, and did not waste time, executing 40,000 Polish Army officers in the Katyn Forest. When the mass graves were discovered, they tried to blame it on the Germans, but irrefutable evidence proved otherwise.

Not much happened on the Western Front during the winter of 1939–40. Some called it the "Phony War." Yet, feverish planning went on among Hitler and the German generals Erich von Manstein, Gerd von Rundstedt, Heinz Guderian, and others during that winter.

At the start of World War II, the Czechs were formally discharged from the Foreign Legion and were transferred to France, to the Czechoslovakian headquarters in Agde, a small Mediterranean village. Still in French uniform, their training continued. The boys lost contact with their parents and Edith in Zilina.

On May 9, 1940, the Germans started the Battle of France with parachute attacks, panzer brigades, and with the *Luftwaffe* against the Netherlands and Belgium. This is when Chamberlain had to resign, and a determined Winston Churchill became the new prime minister, promising pain and suffering to a nation that stood fast with him. The change in the British public was amazing, their endurance heroic. Both the British public and the military suffered enormous losses with gritted teeth and bravery.

The defence of France was in the hands of the nearly seventy-year-old Generalissimo Maurice Gamelin, assisted by the British Expeditionary Forces. Gamelin was found by the

Germans to be outdated, operating with 1914–18 experience and technology. Opposing him was Field Marshal Walther von Brauchitsch, who, although he questioned Nazi ideology, was a first-class professional from an old military family. The Germans had superior equipment and relied heavily on two-way tank-to-tank and Luftwaffe radio contact, which the Allied Forces were lacking.

Gamelin made two fatal mistakes. He put far too many divisions in defence of the Maginot line, opposing the Germans, who had no intention of starting a frontal attack and repeating the trench warfare of the past. Instead, they encircled the French forces. Gamelin also expected a southward turn of the German Army from Belgium. Instead, the German tanks and armoured vehicles passed the Ardennes forest, which the French believed to be "impossible." The result was a disaster.

The Czechoslovak Legion was immediately mobilized, and their convoy left Agde, moving toward Lyons at night, the lorries proceeding without headlights. The Czech army was engaged in battle forty kilometres north of Paris. Laci described in his autobiography how many of the French soldiers had rifles of 1889 issue, single-bullet loading, and some of the ammunition did not fit the chambers. Laci's unit fought the Germans near Columbiers, trying to slow the German advance and cover the retreating French. There was chaos. French soldiers mingling with civilian refugees on the crowded highways made it difficult to perform military operations. Laci's unit moved to Blandureau, then proceeded south of the shore of the Seine, near Montereau. One hindrance in their fight was that the highways were cluttered by pathetic civilians driven by panic. The only way to move was to walk in front of the lorries to clear the way. The sight of the tired, frightened people carrying their bundles was a heartbreaking sight "which will remain in my mind for the rest of my life," wrote Laci.

The retreating French blew the bridge before Laci's unit could cross, with the result that they were now under heavy fire. The farther south their unit moved, the harder the travel became. They reached the town of Gien. Laci was separated from Zolo and Paul. He could see the *Luftwaffe* bombing the city. Soon, the

German planes started to bomb the highways, then, in low flight, indiscriminately machine-gunned the people on the highway. Laci's unit was shooting back with rifles at the low-flying, strafing planes, but the civilians yelled at them, "*Tire pas*, don't shoot!"

The planes left behind a massacre. Corpses lying everywhere; panic ensued. Laci met Paul, but Zolo was nowhere to be found. The unit stopped for one night, then moved all day, staying for another night near Chateauroux, then on a train to Narbone, finally to Sette, a small harbour on the Mediterranean coast. There, they boarded a cargo vessel, which, of course, was immediately overloaded and not at all prepared for transporting that many people. But Laci and Paul also found Uncle Joseph. Zolo was still missing. They finally landed at Plymouth, then continued by train. The unit proceeded to Bristol and settled near Whitchurch.

Laci was surprised by the cheering crowd and singing schoolgirls passing out chocolate to the soldiers. At the Czechoslovakian Legion's headquarters, Laci learned that the Royal Air Force was short of skilled mechanic manpower and was looking for volunteers. With the permission of the Czech Legion, he signed up with the RAF. He took a course where he excelled, and soon was enrolled in a squadron, advancing in rank. The only inconvenience was that they were continuously on the move from airport to airport. Their pride was to service planes to perfection in the shortest time.

Paul remained in the Czechoslovakian Legion and was fighting the Germans in different theatres of war, achieving high rank in his unit.

Uncle Joseph was discharged from the Czech Legion in Whitchurch. He soon befriended a bright, beautiful, local girl, Mary, and it did not take long before they got married. They settled in Whitchurch, and he opened a private rehabilitation and massage clinic, a profession he had learned in Czechoslovakia.

Despite his continuous posting from one airport to another, Laci, too, got married to a British girl, Joyce Breeze, whom he had met at one of the dances held at the hangar, where local girls were welcomed.

Finally, Laci heard about Zolo.

CHAPTER THIRTEEN

Zolo, like Laci and the rest of the boys, was in the Montereau battle, but he was assigned to a different unit, right at the front line. The advancing German soldiers, sheltered by their tank units, were visible to him. They were pouring fire from all directions. Zolo was shooting back but he was unable to see if his rifle fire was effective. Tank shells exploded around him, then the *Luftwaffe* appeared, their bombs falling, dive bombers strafing. Houses collapsed, flames shooting out of their doors and windows. The unceasing artillery fire threw tons of earth into the air. The air was saturated with the smell of explosives, and whining pieces of flying metal could be heard everywhere.

A Czech soldier near Zolo shrieked out and was wounded, bleeding heavily. Zolo grabbed him and, still holding onto his rifle, as he was taught in the Foreign Legion, lifted the body onto his shoulder. The soldier was crying, mumbling in Czech. Finally, Zolo reached a paramedic unit. Zolo was trying to find his way back to his unit when a shell exploded nearby. He felt a strange impact on his left thigh but, strangely, no pain at all. But when he tried to stand up, his leg felt as if it were not his own, and he fell down. Another Czech soldier grabbed Zolo and tossed him onto a passing lorry. It was then that he first felt an enormous pain in his leg. He was dropped off at a nearby hospital, still clutching his rifle till he went blank.

The wound was life-threatening. No, not in a medical sense. The hospital was soon overrun by German soldiers. It was one thing to be a wounded French soldier, and quite another to be a Jewish member of the Czechoslovakian Legion. It was Zolo's good luck that he had retained his Foreign Legion papers as memorabilia. Making use of these documents, he was listed as a member of the French Foreign Legion. After two weeks, he was transported to Oran, then to Sidi-Bel-Abbes, where he was reinstated in the Foreign Legion.

By July, the Vichy government had taken over Southern France and Africa, with Marshal Philippe Petain at the head, as an ally and collaborator of Germany. This meant renewed danger for Zolo, although – at least for a while – he was fairly safe. His job was to cross the Sahara Desert, driving lorries back and forth. And there was another advantage: The Vichy government, as an ally of Germany, made it possible for Zolo to communicate with his parents in Slovakia, another friend of Germany.

Zolo learned of the pitiable situation of his family. The food rationing for Jews was drastically reduced. Aranka made use of her skill as a seamstress to earn a pittance to buy food on the black market. They lived in a small rented room, surrounded by danger. Edith was still working with total devotion as a physician at the forced labour camp. Everyone relied on Edith's physical and mental endurance and on her soothing support of her mates.

Edith got engaged to Valer Glasel, an influential member of the Jewish community who still retained close relations with prominent authority figures. Valer was in a position to get Edith out of the forced labour camp, but she would not hear of it. Her loyalty to her camp companions was such that she refused Valer's repeated offer.

Everything Hugo wrote to Zolo had to be composed "in between the lines" because of Hugo's concern about censors.

After six months of clandestine planning, on June 22, 1941, Hitler attacked the Soviet Union from all the way north to the Black Sea, using several million soldiers and all the power he could muster. This was the famous "Operation Barbarossa," and the Nazis achieved spectacular advances. Soon Ukraine fell, and the *Einsatzgruppe* went to work on the Jewish communities, as well as the local leaders. An estimated one million Jews were killed and buried in mass graves; some were buried still alive, the covering soil over them moving for a while, like in Babi Jar and many other places. The victims included many orthodox Jews from Eastern Slovakia.

On January 20, 1942, a long-planned conference was called at the elegant Wannsee, near Berlin, with Reinhard Heydrich as chairman, who by then was the head of the Czech Protectorate; Adolf Eichmann; Dieter Wisliceny; and other "experts on Jewish affairs." The secret meeting was about the "Final Solution of the Jewish Question" – the technical planning of the Jewish Holocaust; the total elimination of the European Jews. They moved fast, choosing the mode and location of elimination.

A ship, if one can call it that, by the name of *Struma* was chartered by Zionist leaders in Palestine. The intended "illegal" European Jewish immigrants were on the sea for several months but they did reach Istanbul. The Turks argued with the British to allow these people to enter Palestine and deduct their number from the following year's Jewish quota, but they got nowhere. One month after the Wannsee Conference, on February 23, 1942, the Turks towed the crippled ship to the Black Sea, where a Soviet submarine torpedoed it; 768 men, women, and children died. There was one single survivor, who still wanted to go to Palestine. Sir Henry McMahon, the British governor of Palestine, denied entry to him.

The last letter Zolo received from his father was dated April 1942. The Slovaks were enthusiastic about the deportation of the Jews from their territory to Auschwitz, which had just been set up by the Germans. The Slovaks happily paid 500 Reichsmarks to the Germans for each deported Jew, with the condition that "they never come back."

Edith married Valer Glasel. The next morning, Edith and her group were locked in cattle wagons and were on their way to Auschwitz, the brand new "special" camp, as agreed at the Wannsee Conference.

Auschwitz, located in Poland, was not far from Zilina, but their trip was not a priority for the railway. Close to ninety women were herded into each crowded and sealed wagon. Soon, the stench of human bodies was unbearable. Whimpers, sobbing, and squabbles for space filled the metal cage. Edith heard the metal-to-metal squeal of the wheels, and felt the jars and jolts of the starting and stopping wagon, the blasts of the steam brakes, as it gave priority to German troops on their way to the Russian Front. She caught the masculine clamour and holler of the soldiers on the slow-moving train, their radio playing in the darkness, a woman's voice singing, first sounding faint then slowly rising in volume as the train moved closer, the popular song "Lieb Marlene": *"unter der Kaserne bei den grossen Tor, steht eine Laterne . . ."* ("Underneath the lantern by the barrack gate, Darling, I remember the way you used to wait . . .") fading into cadence in the darkness of the night. *Where are they taking us? What does the future bring?* wondered Edith. *And Aranka? Hugo?* There was no answer.

Days later in Zilina, the rest of the Kohns and the Bocks and the remainder of the Jewish community were escorted by merciless Hlinka guards to the brick factory, Tehelna, including the grandmother, Franciska, who was in her eighties, limping on her crutches. Men and women were separated and were locked in different cattle wagons. A Hlinka guard tossed Grandmother's crutches into the freight car after her. Aranka was separated from Hugo, as was Bela from his wife and their seven-year-old, Judith. So was Ilka from her husband and six-year-old son, Ivan.

The youngest Kohn daughter, Elsa, had recently married a widower, Sandor Trossler, who had twin daughters from his first marriage. Magda and Mintika, seven years old, remained the responsibility of Elsa. Mothers with their small children were instantly sent to the gas chambers in Auschwitz. The famous "experiments" with twins by Dr. Mengele had not been set up yet.

Late in 1942, Uncle Zsiga in Budapest received a postcard, mailed in Birkenau, from Uncle Bela. It was a printed script with little squares to be checked off, saying: "I am well; send money; send food," and a return address, which had been a number. It was signed "Bela." Nothing else. Zsiga and Erwin tried to find out where "Birkenau" was located. All their efforts were useless; nobody had heard of the place. Of course, they sent money and food, mainly canned food. Only many years later, when Erwin read William Shirer's book, did he learn that it was the early practice in Auschwitz-Birkenau for inmates to send such cards to relatives abroad, immediately before being gassed.

The time arrived when Zolo was in real danger. No longer was it safe for him to remain under the Nazi Vichy regime. He also felt galvanized to fight the Nazis. The leadership of the Foreign Legion turned out to be his enemy. One day, he escaped; with his small amount of saved money, he got onto an Egyptian cargo ship heading to Portugal. From there, with the help of the captain, he got onto another vessel, which took him to England. He soon located the Czechoslovak Legion and next met Laci in Cardiff. It was a bittersweet reunion. That is when Laci first read Hugo's last letter. Zolo reenlisted in his old unit.

The RAF had just had devastating losses and badly needed new personnel. Zolo volunteered and was "borrowed" by the RAF. After a brief training, Zolo became a tail-gunner in a bomber squadron. He had many dangerous missions over Europe, often doubling as a wireless operator. He met Laci at different times; on some occasions, Laci's squad was servicing his plane. He even once visited Laci's wife, Joyce Breeze, and their baby son, Peter.

It was because of Zolo's mechanical skills that he was chosen for pilot training. He was flown to Montreal (all he could remember of it was the Dorval Airport and a nearby establishment called "Danceland") and to complete his training was sent to Winnipeg.

Back in England, he first flew Vickers Wellingtons, mainly on night missions. Later, he piloted an upgraded form of Liberators. He had far too many missions; he could not recall the exact number, but it was close to sixty. Only on one occasion did Zolo suffer serious damage; his tail-gunner died in combat, and Zolo's landing gear was damaged. Nearing England, he was instructed to throw his bombs, explosives, and excess fuel into the sea. Lots of fire trucks were waiting, and he had a hazardous but lucky landing.

In between Zolo's missions, he visited Laci. The war was slowly coming to an end. All the "borrowed" flyers were returned to the Czech Air Force, which was now fully operational. When the war ended, both Laci and Zolo were assigned to Prague's Ruzyne Airport. Both got two weeks off so that they could visit Zilina.

The only relatives they found there were Uncle Sandor and his wife, Sara, who had just returned from their exile in Hungary to the liberated Slovakia. The sorrow and tears seemed never-ending. They found out that before deportation, Hugo was arrested through the manipulation of an "old friend." In exchange for being "freed," he had to "sell" his house to his betrayer.

Zolo and Laci met some other family friends, who informed them that Hugo had left two suitcases with them with some valuables and family papers, including Edith's university documents.

With heavy heart, they returned to Prague. Laci's only consolation was that his wife, Joyce, had sold the bit of modest furniture they possessed and soon would arrive in Prague with baby Peter.

Then, Laci was called into the office of the commander. Zolo was there, too. Laci learned that Joyce and son Peter had been murdered at their home in England. The news was all over the BBC. Apparently someone who knew that Joyce had some money shot her, and when Peter started crying, he killed him, too.

Laci was a wreck. He had lost all of his family, both old and new. He flew to the burial. Joseph and Mary were waiting for him. At their insistence, Laci remained in their home and, with love and care, was nursed back to life over many months.

CHAPTER FOURTEEN

All hopes now faded for Laci. With heavy heart and deep in sorrow, after some time he found Peggy — or Peggy found him. With her astounding faith and caring, she gently nurtured Laci, and both began to feel a deepening love for one another. Slowly, slowly, once more Laci's life sprouted. They got married and settled in Chester. Soon they had a baby son, Danny, and life was rich again.

Zolo remained in Zilina for a while. He found his old flame from his youth, Vlasta, and they grew close. But for Zolo, Zilina became intolerable, full of memories of his lost family. He could not tell who around him was a friend, if any, or neutral, or enemy. He heard the story that two Hlinka guards got into a fight over a heavy silver candle holder while they were looting Hugo's house, and in the vicious dispute, one shot the other dead. To him, it felt like all around him were murderers.

Most of the Jewish survivors lingered in displaced persons ("DP") camps in Germany. Some who returned to their original countries were received with hostility by the local population, and in some instances, postwar pogroms were sparked, like in Poland and in Hungary.

The American general George S. Patton, a notorious anti-Semite, suggested that all DPs should be deported to Russia, no questions asked. Once, in a military hospital, Patton slapped the face and kicked a soldier suffering from battle fatigue, calling him a "coward." On the verge of being recalled from the European theatre of war, Patton was saved from the humiliation by his bosom friend John McCloy, then U.S. Assistant Secretary of Defense. This is the same McCloy who adamantly refused the repeated request of the leaders of World Jewry, including Golda Meir, to bomb Auschwitz's gas chambers and the railroads leading to Auschwitz. McCloy invented one excuse after another, denying these supplications: "It is too far" – not true, as they were regularly bombing the I.G. Farben factory, thirty kilometres from Auschwitz; "It is the British who decides" – not true; "There are other priorities," etc. His notes to the U.S. Air Force forbidding such bombing missions are preserved in Yad Vashem. McCloy was appointed to be governor of the U.S. Zone of Germany. One of his first priorities was to convert the sentences of Nazi war criminals. For his good deeds, he was awarded honorary German citizenship.

Canada's border was still closed to Jews. The British continued to prevent Jewish immigration to Palestine, while they eagerly trained and armed the Transjordanian Legion. One "illegal" ship, the *Exodus*, left for Palestine from the French port of Sette in mid-July 1947 with 4,515 Holocaust survivors. An armada of British warships attacked them in international waters. Three Jews died in the violent boarding of the ship. Despite British demands, the French refused to reaccept them, unless the passengers wished to do so. Of course, they did not. The British then deported these Holocaust survivors back to Germany and, while the UN and the international press witnessed it, they attacked the ship with hundreds of their soldiers and military police. Many men and women were injured, and the survivors were forced into barbed wire-surrounded "camps," under the authority of a German commander and German guards to watch over them. It was around that time that the United Kingdom ordered Canada's borders to be opened for Jewish immigration (they had the power to do so under the British–North America Act), in order to relieve the pressure for Jewish immigration to Palestine.

It was then that Zolo and Vlasta decided to immigrate to the newly established Israel. They wanted to be in the midst of their own. Zolo told Erwin his story. Zolo and Vlasta arrived at Haifa by ship early in the morning. Israel's War of Liberation was then in progress. On disembarking, everyone was asked what their profession may be. Zolo said that he was a pilot. They were immediately driven to the military headquarters, and the same evening he was in Zagreb, Yugoslavia. He had to pick up Czech armaments and personnel. His plane was so overloaded, he had difficulty gaining altitude.

Thereafter, Zolo was in the Israeli Air Force, where he remained for the rest of his life. He fought in the Israeli War of Liberation and in other campaigns that followed. In 1950, he showed his Cousin Erwin a small lot, at the time still somewhat of a desert, covered with red sand, in Zahala, not far from Tel Aviv, where a modest family home was built for him by the Israeli Air Force. One of his neighbours was Yitzhak Rabin, later his tennis partner. He used to fly a rickety Dakota to Eilat twice weekly, where Erwin worked as a physician. In those days, Eilat had a population of four hundred people and no electricity.

Zolo became a father. First a boy, also called Danny, was born, then a girl, Anat.

One winter's night, Zolo was driving home. The rain came down in huge, heavy drops, typical of the Israeli rainy season. At one of the crossroads, he spotted a woman, wet through and through, her outstretched hand and closely held fingers begging to be picked up. Zolo hesitated. He did not like to pick up anybody, particularly women, at night. But in the downpour, he felt sorry for the dripping wet creature. He gave her a ride and turned on the heater. He did not suspect the drama to come.

The woman was grateful, of course, and thanked Zolo with poor Ivrit (Hebrew) but with a familiar accent. She was in her forties and she was from Slovakia.

She, too, found Zolo's Ivrit to be less than perfect, heavily accented. "Where are you from?" the woman inquired, suspecting the answer.

"From Slovakia."

"I can tell that from your accent. Which part of Slovakia?" she asked again.

"Zilina."

"And your name?" Zolo hesitated.

"Zolo Bock," he said finally.

With that, the woman started to cry and wail.

"What is the matter?" a startled Zolo asked.

"Did you have a sister, Edith?"

Now it was Zolo's turn to be shocked. "Yes, indeed," he said. The car slowed down.

"I am alive because of Edith! I know what happened to Edith and your mother," the woman said, sobbing.

Zolo had to pull the car to the side of the road and stop. Still suspicious, he asked his passenger: "What did you say?"

"I was in Auschwitz in 1942. Your sister Edith worked in a small hospital which was set up for the Kapos [Kamp Polizei]. The Kapos were Jews, but as bad as the Nazis."

"How come you remember my sister after so many years?" asked an astonished Zolo.

"Wait," cried the woman. "When Edith arrived at Auschwitz in early July 1942, a bunch of girls piped up, 'She is our physician!' The Kapo took Edith into an office, and the next thing Edith knew, she was assigned to work in the small hospital set up for the Kapos. But she constantly watched for her mother to arrive. Soon her mother's transport arrived; I don't recall her name."

"Aranka," said Zolo.

"That's it. Edith begged the Kapo to let her have a nurse's aide. Edith thought that would be safer for her mother. All was fine till December fifth, 1942. Then, Edith's mother was chosen for a lineup. Everyone knew that it was for the gassing. Edith went crazy."

"How do you know this? How come you remember?"

"Wait. I was in the lineup for the gassing myself, on my way to death. Edith suddenly sneaked up to the line, grabbed me, gave me a push, and took my place. The group did not move for a while yet. Edith hugged her mother. 'What is your name?' I asked her from a safe distance. 'Edith Bock from Zilina,' said she. 'Who is she?' I inquired from the others of the hospital staff.

"Then came Edith's last words: 'If you find Valer Glasel, tell him that I loved him.' Then I pulled away. And that is why I am alive today. Edith chose to go to the gas with her mother."

Zolo was numb. He sat in the car motionless for a long time. Then he drove the woman to the house where she lived. Zolo took her name and telephone number. The rain kept pattering on the top of the car, Zolo's tears running down his face. Then, still sobbing, he drove home.

But Israel is full of strange stories like that.

EPILOGUE

For countless years, my Cousin Edith's chronicle never left my mind. I did write her story once in my autobiography, but the way I described it there reflected the bare facts only — the skeleton of the events, so to speak — but failed to introduce her daily life and her character, as I have known Edith.

Yet it always remained my intention to bring Edith back to life, as she used to be, as I knew her, even for such a short while. I could not bear the thought that only a small pile of ashes, if anything, remained of her somewhere on the windswept fields near Auschwitz. I lost twenty-four close relatives in the Holocaust. I mourn each of them with deep sorrow, for each had a remarkable story.

But the loss of Edith has endured, and still languishes after all these years. I cannot account for why I was wounded so deeply by Edith's doom. Could it be because she was a medical student when I, as a child, just dreamed to enter the same demanding profession? Maybe because fate has ordained that our stories would have so many similarities? Maybe because our medical studies, beyond our control, had been interrupted in the last year of our studies — all examinations written — by evil political forces, hers by the Nazis, mine by the Soviets? Maybe because I felt the same pain from a lost hope? But, unlike Edith, I was lucky. Following similar paths, I found opportunities to complete my studies. True, due to circumstances, I had to write all my examinations three times, in Hungarian, German, and English. Maybe because I, too, faced imminent death by impending execution on the shore of the Danube together with a pregnant wife?

All these years, Edith has never left my mind. Far from

being a poet, I wrote two poems for her, some twenty years ago, one in English, the other in Latin.

To Edith

You have been my Mentor,
My first honoured Preceptor,
My beloved cousin and Magister,
Auld Prague's Alumna,
Famulus of Celsus, Aesculap's recruit,
With sweet smile, blonde hair on your brow.

Your days were hard labour, I know what it takes!
—Set aside pleasure, negate the play
Toil and study while long years will pass—
Your dream almost fulfilled but at what a price!

Happiness rarely touched your girlish face,
Your worriless days were but a few,
Just-now wed bride, your marital bliss
Lasted a single day,
Then torn away, away forever!

Is there a way to make you say,
Invite you to whisper a message?
My murdered Lambkin, colleague and cousin
Your life was stolen away!

So long ago now, you stood there in awe
Mothering your frightened-sick mother,
In the cursed pyre, in devouring fire
Auschwitz's ovens consumed you all!

Shema Yisroel, I won't see again
Your maidenly smile, dear honey blonde cousin,
Alav Ha' Shalom, may you rest in peace,
El Molei Rachamim.

To Edith Again – *Denuo ad* Edith

Requiscat in pace
Consubrina dulce,
Ego recordo nominem tuam
In aeternam memoriam.

Requiescat in pace
Consubrina benedicta,
Doctor medicinae, nostra Edith
Cum capello aureo
Quisquis tantum pacit.

I hadn't been in Prague during Edith's student years, in her beloved city. I had the knowledge of the deep cultural treasures of the Czech culture; I had known about the joys and the struggles and daily life of students in three continents. But I had no direct knowledge of Edith's daily life in Prague. Wishing to see her thrive again, I had to invent her life in Prague, her circle of friends. I could not know Edith's examination questions, so I substituted them with mine. But her professors, the historic facts, the composers, writers, are real persons who did exist in Prague. The Domoj ("home" in Czech) is the prototype of students' restaurants that exist in every university city.

I needed many sources to refresh my mind about the spelling of some names, historic personages, and exact dates. For that, Laci's unpublished autobiography, countless discussions with Zolo, and the Internet were extremely useful tools, as were different sources. In particular, Zolo's accidental meeting with the woman Edith had saved while sacrificing herself, and the facts of Edith's last days in Auschwitz, I learned from my Cousin Zolo. I obtained some precious original family documents, including Edith's University Report Book, from Zolo's daughter, Anat Bock-Grosz, Zahala, Israel.

My writing has been frequently interrupted with bitter tears and sorrow. But it also gave me the satisfaction of bringing Edith back to life!

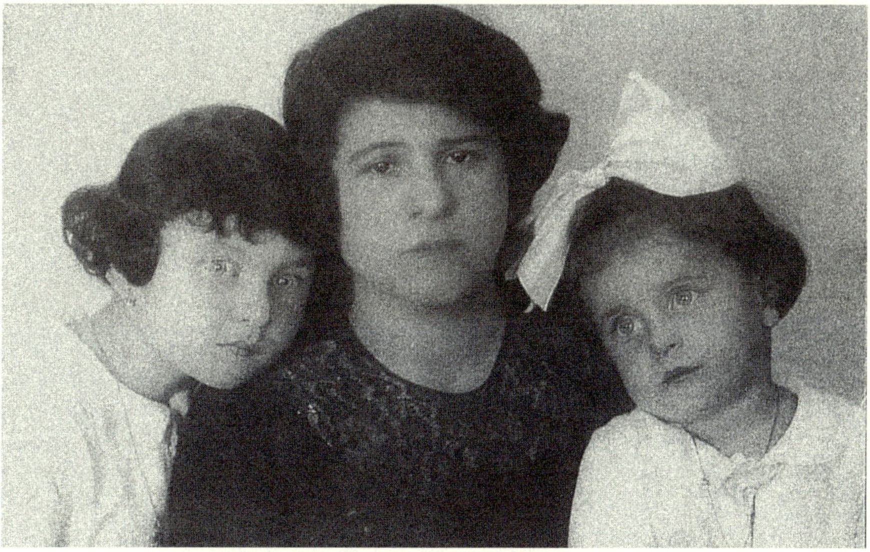

Elsa with the twins Magda and Mintika

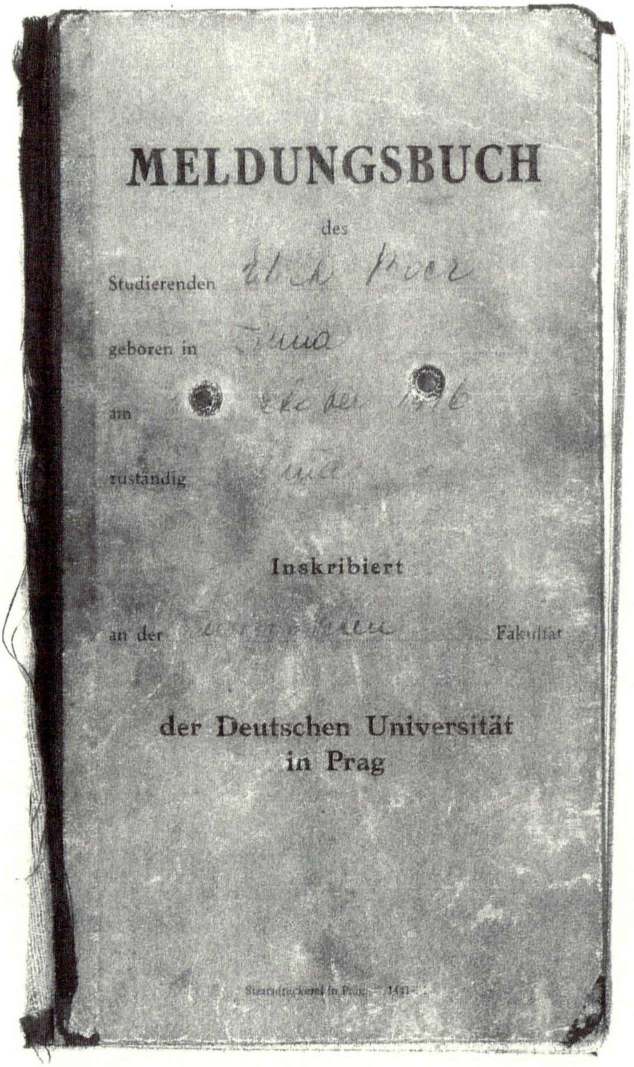

MELDUNGSBUCH

des

Studierenden

geboren in

am

zuständig

Inskribiert

an der Fakultät

der Deutschen Universität
in Prag

Edith's university document.

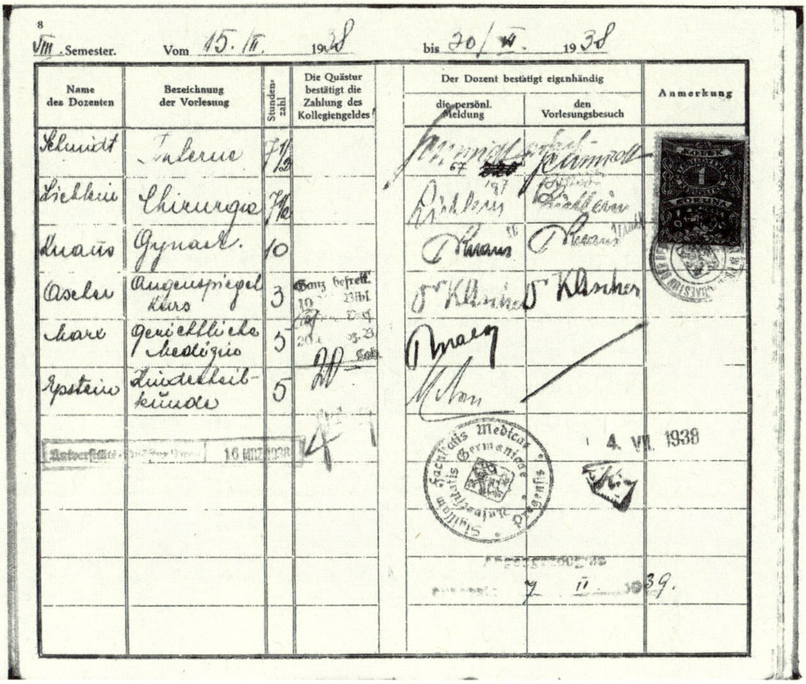

8

VIII. Semester. Vom 15. III. 1938 bis 30/VI. 1938

Name des Dozenten	Bezeichnung der Vorlesung	Stundenzahl	Die Quästur bestätigt die Zahlung des Kollegiengeldes	Der Dozent bestätigt eigenhändig: die persönl. Meldung	den Vorlesungsbesuch	Anmerkung
Schmidt	Interne	7½				
Schloffer	Chirurgie	7½		Schloffer	Schloffer	
Knaus	Gynaek.	10		Knaus	Knaus	
Ascher	Augenspiegelkurs	3	Ganz befreit. 10 Bibl. ... 20 Sek.	Dr Klinker	Dr Klinker	
Marx	Gerichtliche Medizin	5		Marx		
Epstein	Kinderheilkunde	5				

16 MRZ 1938

4. VII. 1938

Sigillum Facultatis Medicae Universitatis Germanicae Pragensis

7. II. 1939.

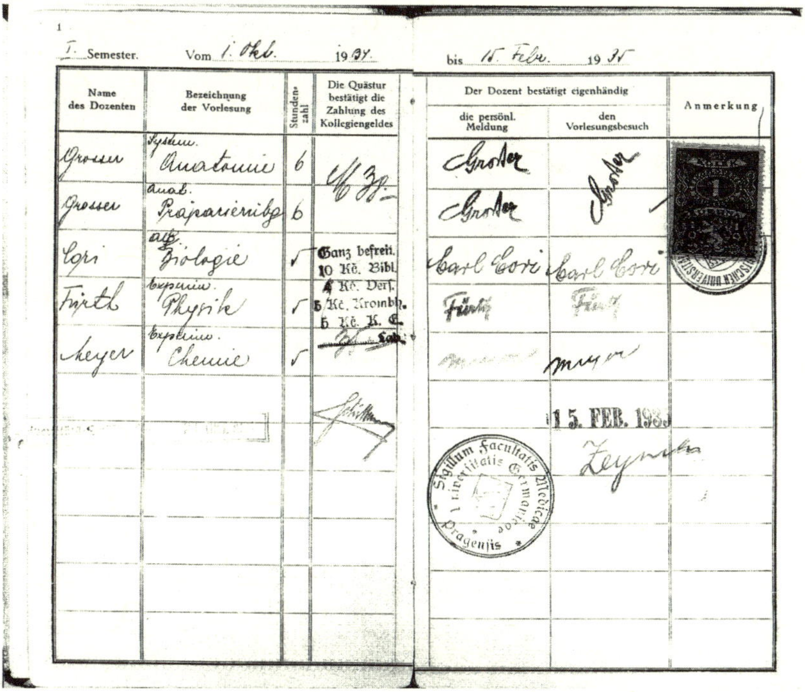

1

I. Semester. Vom 1. Okt. 1934. bis 15. Febr. 1935

Name des Dozenten	Bezeichnung der Vorlesung	Stundenzahl	Die Quästur bestätigt die Zahlung des Kollegiengeldes	Der Dozent bestätigt eigenhändig: die persönl. Meldung	den Vorlesungsbesuch	Anmerkung
Grosser	System. Anatomie	6		Grosser	Grosser	
Grosser	anat. Präparierübg	6		Grosser		
Cori	allg. Biologie	5	Ganz befreit. 10 Kč. Bibl. 4 Kč. Vers. 5 Kč. Krankh. 5 Kč. K. C.	Carl Cori	Carl Cori	
Fürth	experim. Physik	5		Fürth	Fürth	
Meyer	experim. Chemie	5			Meyer	

15. FEB. 1935

Sigillum Facultatis Medicae Universitatis Germanicae Pragensis

Žilina dňa 22. IV. 1940

Moji drahí !!

Neopisatlenou radostou sme od Vás dnes dva dopisi obdržali, a tešíme sa že sa Vám dobre ve - die.

Veď naša najväčšia starost, len to je, či sa dobre máte, a či netrpíte skrze dnešnej situacie.

Chcem Vám teraz o všetkom napísať, čo je u nás nového a starého.

1./ všetci sme zdraví, a sme všetci spolu, ako sme aj boli.

2./ obchod ešte dalej tak máme, ako aj predošle. Aj tovaru máme ešte viac ako predtím, lebo som tich pár korun čo mi samu ostalo, tiež do tovaru investoval. Väčšia chiba je to, že teraz ništ netržime. Vtedi keď sme nemali tovaru, tak bi sa bol predal, a dnes keď ho máme až po krky tak nik nekupuje.

3./ ako som Vám uš bol napísal, sme sa sbytom prestahovali, vedla obchodu na I. poschodie kde niekedi Hugo Linzenberg mal obchod. Tento dom kupil Osadský krajčír, a uncho bívame.

Aj Marci a Ilka sa museli prestahovať, bivaleho našeho domu. Ilka ešte vždi preváďža obchod sdáždnikami, veď sa stoho najviac udržuje.

4./ Žuža 30 marca 1940 išla do Palestíny, a ako sme obdržali správu uš aj štastlive tam došla.

Starí rodičia mali tiež velku radost, keď sme jim Vaše dva listy prečítali.

Radi bi sme raz jeden list obdržali, vktorom sa aj deti podpísané.

Inač je u nás dosial všetko pri starom, jak dlho budeme mať tento pokoj neviem, lebo stále riešia tu židovsku otázku.

Aj Katka s Prievidzi išla pred 8 dnami do Palestíni.

Stímtom transportom išli aj zo Žiliny asi 30 osoby, medzinima aj Hugo Linzenberg. Ale ako sa dozvedáme, uš 8-10 dni trčia na lode v Bratislave a ani sem ani tam.

Maju nejaké prekážky s lodou, tak že ešte stále nevedno či odijdu alebo nie.

Feri sa stále tak má ako aj pred rokom. Raz sa mu lepšie vedie, a raz horšie.

Sme sa uš radovali, že Editku na tento smester zoberu na universitu, a ostatnej chvíle nám to pokazili, tak že znovu musí čekat na príležitost, kedi može dokončit.

Prosíme Vás uprímne napíšte nám zaraz znovu, lebo to je naša jedinná radost, keď od Vás dobre správi dostaneme.

Tento mesiac 12. Apríla mala maminka Geburtstag, tak som jej vo vašom mene dva peknie kvetini kupil, a Vaše vizitky priležil, takže keď kvetinár doniesol kvety, skoro sa rozplakala pred radostou.

Dnes máme sederabend, nemá kto u nás máništanu modliť.

Uš nemám Vám čo dalej napísať. Prajem Vám aj na dalej čo najlepšie zdravie a mnoho štastie.

Buďte všetci od nás mnohokrát boskávaní a pozdravení

Hugo Aranka a Edith

[illegible]

Hugo's letter from Zilna to his sons in North Africa. Spring 1940.

[Letter translated by Zolo]

My Dears, Zilina, 22.4.1940

I cannot describe our joy on receiving today your tow letters.
We are happy to hear that you are well, since our greatest worry is whether you are well and whether you do not suffer from the present situation.
Now I want to write to you about everything new and old.
1.We are all of us healthy and together as we were before.
2.We still have the store as before. We have merchandise even a bigger stock than before because the few crowns which were left I invested in the stock. The bigger problem is that now we do not sell. When we did not have merchandise we could have sold. Today when we have it up to our necks, nobody buys.
3.As I had written we moved from our appartment to the first floor beside our store, where once in the past Hugo Liazenberg had his business. This house was bought by the Community taylor and we live on his property. Marci and Ilka had to move from our house as well. Ilka still runs her business with umbrellas as that is her main incom.
4.Zuza left for Palestine on the 30 of March and we have already received news of her successful arrivel. Grandparents were happy as well when we read to them your tow letters. We would be happy to receive one letter with the childrens signitures. Apart from that everything is here as before, how long we will have this quite break I do not know because all the time they are bussy solving the jewish question. Also Katka from Prievidze left 8 days ago to Palestian. With this transport from Zilina went 30 people and among them Hugo Linzenberg, but we are now imformed that they are stuck in Bratislava and nither here nor there. There is some obstacle arownd the boat so that it is still not clear whether they leave or stay.
Feri gets on as he did a year ago, sometimes better, sometimes worse.
We were happy that Editka was accepted for this semester at the University but at the last minute they cancelled it so now again she has to wait for the opportunity to be able to finish.
We ask you sincerely write to us again because this is our only joy, when we get good news of you.
This mounth on April 12 maminka had her birthday, so in your name I bought two beautiful flowers and added your visit cards, when the delivery boy bruught the flowers she nearly cried from joy.
Today we have the "Seder" evening and there is no one to pray the "Manishtana"
I have nothing more to write about. I wish you continuous good health and the best of luck. Be many times kissed by all of us and with best regards,

Hogo Aranka and Edith

If it is possible send us a picture of you so that we can see you at least that way.

Translation of Hugo's letter on opposite page.

THE HOLOCAUST VICTIMS OF ŽILINA

(Updated on the 29th of June 2003)

Ableser Samuel	Axelrad Klára	Berkovič Irma
Ableser Ružena	Back Alžbeta	Better Jozef
Ableser Bernát	Back Anna	Better Malvina
Ableser Margita	Back Michal	Better Gejza
Adler Helena	Balint Teodor	Biel Adolf
Adler Antonia	Balint Šarolta	Biel Jozef
Adler Žigmund	Bán Imrich	Biel Berta
Adler Magdalena	Baumhorn Anna	Biel Klára
Adler Alica	Baumhorn Margita	Bielik Alžbeta
Adler Jakub	Baumhorn Pavel	Bielik Ivan
Adler Julia	Baumhorn Junta	Bielik Ruth
Adler Armin	Baumhorn Paula	Birnbaum Lota
Adler Edita	Baumhorn Mária	Birnbaum Miriam
Adler Roland	Baumhorn Arnošt	Birnbaum Róbert
Adler Julia	Baumhorn Edita	Blau Moric
Adler Jozef	Baumhorn Erika	Blau Ervin
Adler Leo	Beck Františka	Blau Alica
Adler Eugen	Beim Henrik	Blau Marianna
Adler Hermina	Beim Leontina	Blau Margita
Adler Eva	Beim Nathan	Blau Hanna
Alt Mariena	Beim Malvina	Blauhorn Milan
Alt František	Berényi Samuel	Blauhorn Flora
Alt Viliam	Berényi Rozalia	Blaum Irma
Altmann Koloman	Berényi Ružena	Blitz Šara
Altmann Cecilia	Berényi Eugen	Blüh Maximilian
Altmann Robert	Berényi Renáta	Blüh Irena
Altmann Blanka	Berényi Jolana	Blüh Kurt
Altmann Pavel	Berényi Vojtech	Blüh Juraj-Tomaš
Altmann Ida	Berényi Hermina	Blüh Ludovit
Altmann Samuel	Berényi Arpád	Blüh Anna
Altmann Róza	Berényi Arnold	Blüh Erika
Altmann Marcel Dr.	Berényi Gizela	Blüh Karol
Altmann Robert-Poldi	Berger Samuel	Blüh Klotilda
Apfelmann Valeria	Berger Janka	Blüh Štefania
Apotheker Jozef	Berger Gizela	Blüh Artur
Apte Michal	Berger Šarolta	Blüh Imrich
Apte Olga	Berger Ida	Blüh Vojtech Michal
Arimovič Leo	Berger Armin Ing.	Blüh Zita
Arimovič Augustina	Berger Izidor	Bock Edita
Auerbach Richard	Berger Magda	Bock Hugo
Auerbach Margita	Berger Jozef	Bock Aranka
Auerbach Evelina	Bergsmann Adolf	Bock Marcel
Auerbach Edita	Berkovič Anna	Bock Helena
Auerbach Arnošt	Berkovič Adolf	Bock Ivan

Sources

Bock, Laci. *Autobiography*. Unpublished, n.d.

Elon, Amos. *The Pity of It All: A Portrait of the German-Jewish Epoch*. New York: Henry Holt & Co., 2003.

Gordon, Haim. *The Rise and Decline of the Jewish Community of Zilina*. Translated from Hebrew by Elisabeth Meier–Weil and Zuzka Weil. Jerusalem: Self-published, 2003. [Describes the history of the Jews in Zilina in 31 pages and, additionally, 2,668 Holocaust victims listed alphabetically, including Edith, Aranka, Hugo, and the entire Bock and Kohn family.]

Koranyi, Erwin K. *Dreams and Tears: Chronicle of a Life*. Renfrew, Ontario: General Store Publishing House, 2006.

Loftus, John, and Mark Aarons. *The Secret War against the Jews: How Western Espionage Betrayed the Jewish People.* New York: St. Martin's Press, 1990.

Morse, Arthur D. *While Six Million Died: A Chronicle of American Apathy*. New York: The Overlook Press, 1983.

Shirer, William L. *The Rise and Fall of the Third Reich: A History of Nazi Germany*. New York: Simon & Schuster, 1990.

About the Author

Erwin K. Koranyi, M.D., F.R.C.P. (c), Professor Emeritus of Neuropsychiatry at the University of Ottawa, was born in Budapest, Hungary, in 1924. He was dedicated to being a physician since his early childhood. He survived the Holocaust with great losses and pain, then escaped from a choking Soviet rule to the West after a few years. In the midst of post-war poverty, he graduated in Medicine in Innsbruck, Austria.

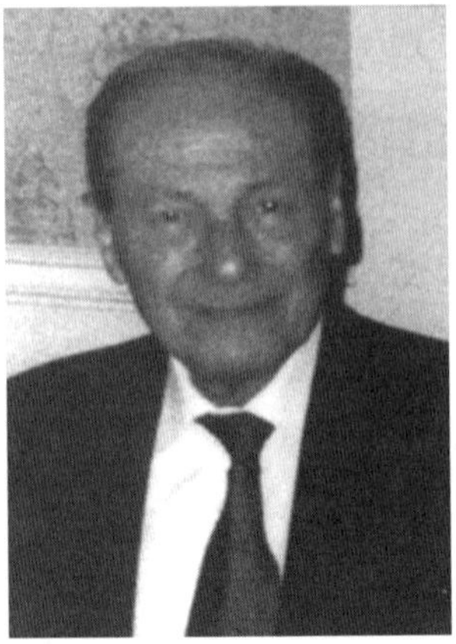

Dr. Koranyi was chief of the Psychiatric Outpatient Unit at the Ottawa General Hospital, then was Director of Education and head of a neuropsychiatric unit at the Royal Ottawa Hospital. He also established an International Course of Psychiatry at the University of Ottawa. His early writings ran along professional lines: two books and fifty-five articles, published in refereed journals.

It took him many years to process his early life under the Nazi regime in Hungary and to write his autobiography (*Dreams and Tears*), as well as to produce this current book. His other stories, poems, and essays remain unpublished.